CELIAC DISEASE:
A Chronology of Calamities & Celebrations

Ron W. Webster

Copy editing by Kathleen E. Huycke

Published by Ron W. Webster
2016

First Printing: 2016

ISBN 978-1-365-22439-3

Ron W. Webster
P.O. Box 401-430 Webb Place
Winnipeg, Manitoba R3B 3J7

www.books-ron-w-webster.com

To my lovely wife Kathleen for her constant support, love and devotion, and to my very caring sister Elaine, my late brother Dennis, my cousin Ray Aikens and my good friend Randy Clark, all who stuck with me through my darkest hours and continue throughout to celebrate our lives together.

Thank you. Without your support and patience, I truly believe I would not have the strength to continue onward.

Table of Contents

PREFACE

This book is an account of my life with celiac disease. I was diagnosed in an era when very little was known about celiac disease and there were no commercially produced gluten free food products or baking ingredients available. How does one survive without bread, pasta, cereal and all those common foods containing gluten? What happens when one cannot find gluten free food and continues to eat foods containing gluten?

Being very animate about this issue, I have advocated for several years by means volunteering with the Canadian Celiac Association (CCA) as newsletter publisher for several years. Although I am NOT a public speaker, I was asked to tell my story at a CCA Conference to a group of newly diagnosed celiac patients and to a group of registered dietitians. Afterwards, I was approached by several parents to express they had not considered the dangers for their children to be tempted by peer pressure to "have a burger or pizza" with their friends. One elderly lady came up to me and bluntly stated, "Your speech was very informative, we need more people like you". I was very flattered indeed, but she quickly sprinted away before I could tell her that my whole agenda is to prevent people like me!

My advice to anyone with celiac disease is to join a support group like the Canadian Celiac Association. As a member you will find support, camaraderie and learn much about celiac disease which will only make your life so much better. Personally, as a member of the Manitoba Chapter, I have gained much insight into the issue and am much healthier for it today.

I invite you to have a rather intimate look at my life of medical calamities, miraculous recoveries and all the celebrations of a life that has, at times, teetered on the brink of death.

CHAPTER ONE

Where it All Began

I came into the world in 1949, on January 9th at about 1:30 am. My family consisted of my Mother, Father and two brothers; Ken who was age seven and Dennis who was age five at the time. When it was time to leave the hospital (St. Boniface General), my parents took me home to Egerton Road in St. Vital.

Of course I do not remember much of my life for the first two or three years, but I do have a few tidbits that are worthy of mention.

Memories of life on Egerton Road.

One of the first fiascos I have some recollection of is the day Dennis and Ken blew the mailbox off the wall of the house. Ken had gotten some blockbuster fireworks from somewhere and being an adventurous one, he suggested to Dennis they see what would happen if they put a lit one in the mailbox. Well we all found out! All I heard was a big bang and the mailbox fell to the ground with such a clamor our Mom came running out to see what the commotion was. Of course Ken and Dennis were nowhere to be seen and I was standing there all alone to face the wrath of Mom!

Next to our home on Egerton road was a mini forest. It is still there but somewhat smaller now. Ken and Dennis had built a fort in the bush and one day Ken, Dennis and I were playing in the fort when they decided to make a fire. The fire got out of hand and burned most of the fort and some surrounding bush. Luckily they had some water and blankets to beat out the fire and managed to put the fire out. Ken and Dennis made me promise to not tell Mom, and I vowed my allegiance to my brothers. I'm happy to say it wasn't me that squealed this time, it was Dennis! Apparently Dennis had nightmares about the fire and was talking in his sleep about it. Mom heard this and in the morning asked Dennis what he was dreaming about last night. Of course Dennis denied everything, as did Ken. So when Mom turned to me, I fidgeted about while looking down to the ground; after all, I did plead allegiance, but Mom is all powerful! Mom decided to give me reprieve and went out to the fort to see for herself. When she returned, we were all grounded for one month. Mom declared, "No one was allowed in the bush for one month."

One other vivid memory I have of my life on Egerton Road is that at about four or five years old, I asked my Mom if I could meet my brothers at Glenwood School and walk back home with them. The school was about two blocks from our home on Egerton Road and I had walked there a few times with Mom and Dennis, so Mom felt I would be safe and said yes. It was in the winter time so I was warmly dressed and set out with my Flyer wagon to meet Ken and Dennis. I wasn't until I was approached by two ladies who were dressed in long black "dresses" and were wearing black veils with "white hats and bibs" that I realized I was lost. (Later I learned the ladies were nuns and to this day have the utmost respect for them.) The ladies asked me where I was going and I said, "I am going to meet my brothers at school". It was obvious to them that I was lost because it was dark out. They asked, "Where do you live?" I looked around but didn't see anything familiar so I replied, "I don't know". They took me to a store and one lady asked if she could use the phone and the other lady bought me a drink and a chocolate bar. After talking on the phone, the lady came over and said there are some nice men coming to take you home. When the men got there, the two ladies hugged me and said goodbye. The two men were dressed in uniforms and drove a car with a red light on the roof. They put me in the car and my wagon in the trunk and started driving. As we were driving one of the men told me my Mom was really worried about me. I asked him if he knew my Mom and he said, "She called him because she could not find you". He explained that they were police officers and that Mom asked them to find me and take me back home. I was afraid Mom would be upset with me but when we arrived home my Mom, Dad, Dennis and Ken were all in tears. When I got out of the car Mom came running to me with open arms.

It wasn't until many years later that Dennis told me how upset Mom was about me being lost. He told me that there were tracks down to the (Seine) river and a hole in the ice. He recounted that the police came and found that a dog had broken through the ice and reported this to Mom. It must have been terrifying time for my Mom, Dad and brothers.

A life changing event and medical diagnosis.

On April 6th, 1954, our baby sister, Elaine, came on the scene. I don't recall much about the events at but shortly after Elaine was born we were both admitted into the Children's Hospital. Apparently we had similar symptoms; (I wasn't aware of any "symptoms"). I do recall one or two events during our stay in the hospital which I believe was probably four or five days.

One event involved a nurse wielding what I perceived to be a "giant" needle. If memory serves me she poked my finger with this "giant" needle and it really hurt! Then the nurse walked toward Elaine who was in the same room in a crib. I said to the nurse, "Don't hurt my sister".

During our stay in the hospital we were fasting. Finally one day they brought Elaine a bottle and me a tray of food. I was really hungry and began eating when suddenly the lady that brought the tray ran over to me and said, "I gave you the wrong tray" and replaced it with a bowl of jelly! What a disappointment. I was hungry and just wanted to go home!

We finally went home and soon found that Mom was giving us strange food we had never had before and not letting us eat bread, cake, cookies and all kinds of stuff. Mom explained that it was because the other food makes us sick so we could not eat it anymore. We were diagnosed with celiac disease.

I believe our parents were told that we could not eat any foods containing gluten which were wheat, rye and barley. Also on the list of foods we could not eat were chocolate and fats of any kind (including fried foods, butter and even milk). Eventually it was discovered that chocolate and fats were not the cause of celiac symptoms and were removed from the list of forbidden foods. Thank goodness chocolate isn't restricted!

What is celiac disease?

Celiac disease (also called celiac sprue or gluten-sensitive enteropathy) is a digestive disease that damages the small intestine and interferes with absorption of nutrients from food. People who have celiac disease cannot tolerate a protein called gluten, found in wheat, rye and barley.

When people with celiac disease eat foods containing gluten, their immune systems respond by damaging the small intestine. This injury occurs to tiny finger like protrusions, called villi, which line the small intestine, and are critical in allowing absorption of nutrients and preventing malnutrition.

Because the body's own immune system causes the damage, celiac disease is considered an autoimmune disorder. However, it is also classified as a disease of malabsorption because nutrients are not absorbed, as well as a genetic disease, meaning it runs in families.

What are the complications associated with celiac disease?

Damage to the small intestine and the resulting nutrient absorption put people with celiac disease at risk for malnutrition and anemia. Other less common associated risks include: Osteoporosis, a condition in which bones become brittle and are at risk for fracture; menstrual and reproductive issues including miscarriage and infertility; short stature, which can occur when childhood celiac disease prevents nutrient absorption; seizures; and cancers such as lymphoma and adenocarcinoma of the small intestine.

In addition, people with celiac disease may often have other autoimmune diseases such as thyroid disease, systemic lupus erythematosus (SLE), Type I diabetes, inflammatory bowel disease, rheumatoid arthritis, Sjogren's syndrome, or collagen vascular diseases. These diseases may require additional testing.

www.asge.org

CHAPTER TWO

A New Beginning

A move to the country.

Our next memorable adventure was moving to Elkhorn, Manitoba in 1955. Elkhorn is located in Westman on the Trans-Canada Highway about 10 miles (16 kilometers) from the Saskatchewan border. My parents purchased a house and a welding and repair business in Elkhorn which became "Webster's Welding & Repair".

The family car was a 1949 Ford Prefect. The Prefect is a small British made car. It had these quaint little arms that popped out from the side of the car when the turn signal was activated. This little car was packed when all six of us were jammed into it.

Dad drove, Mom sat next to Dad with Elaine on her lap, Ken and Dennis sat on the back seat and I sat on the floor under Dennis' legs with my back against the door. I recall as we drove down Portage Avenue the city seemed to end at Polo Park. As we continued west into the current day Westwood, I noticed a building with a mural of a tall tramp and the words "54 miles to Portage" and "It's a long Tramp". That mural has been maintained over the years and is still displayed on the building.

This mural is located at 2579 Portage Avenue and is Winnipeg's oldest known Mural. It has been a city landmark for decades, with an origin that dates back to the 1920's. http://themuralsofwinnipeg.com

Somewhere along the Trans-Canada Highway, as I was leaning on the back door of the Prefect, the door opened and I found myself watching the pavement go by. Dennis immediately grabbed my arm and yelled at me to hang on while Dad retorted from the driver's seat, "Settle down back there". Dennis told Dad that the door came open so Dad quickly pulled over to the side of the highway and stopped. Dad soon had the door fixed and instructed us to make sure the door is locked and don't bump the door handle.

Exploring our new home.

Finally we made it to Elkhorn and as we drove into the driveway at the front of our new home Mom was excited. It was a large brick house with a beautiful big bay window extending from the living room. We entered the house from the back door that lead directly into a huge kitchen; from there we explored the adjacent living room with the big bay window. Mom immediately made plans that violets, geraniums and ferns were going to occupy this space and thrive here, and she was absolutely right. Mom's plants were bountiful and a beautiful addition to the living room. Across the hall from the living room was another room a little smaller than the living room. The upstairs boasted one large bedroom plus 3 smaller bed rooms. There was an additional room at the back side of the house which was empty; this would be our future bathroom.

The move to Elkhorn was probably the riskiest venture my parents ever attempted. Dad's uncle lived in Elkhorn and advised him of a welding/repair business for sale in Elkhorn, and of potential opportunities available due to the "oil boom" in nearby Virden and surrounding area.

One of Dad's multi talents was welding. He obtained certification as a welder at Manitoba Institute of Technology. His plan was to obtain spin-off repair and fabrication work from the pipeline and oil fields.

CHAPTER THREE

Life in Elkhorn

Getting down to business.

Everything appeared to be going well as we settled into an entirely different lifestyle from that of Winnipeg. Dad built a reputation of quality workmanship that was delivered on time at a fair price and was kept quite busy. Dad also did repair and welding projects for local farmers and contractors.

Then the "boom bust"! The oil fields began to dwindle as evidenced by the following quote:

"By the late 1950's, in spite of an increase in the number of producing wells, the oil fields were being operated under natural depletion and field production began to decline. The 1957 production of 16,000 barrels per day had decreased to 10,300 barrels per day in 1963".

Virden ~ Review 19S7 - 1970 Published in 1970 by Virden Town Council

Owing to the downturn of oil production, local farmers and contractors became his main customer base which resulted in a reduction of revenue and eventually lead to our return to Winnipeg.

Adapting to our new surroundings.

As for our home life, it was different from that in Winnipeg, to say the least. Our new home did not have the conveniences of our Egerton Road home. It had no running water, bathroom or source of heat.

For the first few months, until Dad installed a well and pump, we had to get buckets of water from our kindly neighbors, the Watsons. We bathed in a galvanized tub with water we had to carry from the Watsons and heat on the stove. Needless to say, bath day was a big undertaking considering there were six of us. Once Dad had the water system installed, his next project was a bath tub. He built a small room in one corner of the kitchen to house the bathtub. (I now understand why Dad installed the bathtub in the kitchen; the room on the second floor was not structurally sound for a big heavy tub full of water. So now we had the beginnings of a bathroom, but not yet a toilet.

Speaking of toilets, have you ever trudged fifty yards out into the dark in mid-winter to an outhouse? That was a real memorable experience and I can assure you we did not doddle when doing our business! Before the second winter, Dad had built a toilet in the unused upstairs room. It was composed of a wooden box which accommodated a five gallon pail with a toilet seat. Now we can enjoy the luxury of (semi-modern) conveniences once again!

Our home was heated with two stoves in which we burned wood and or coal, which ever was available. This created another task which was assigned to us kids. Ken being the oldest was the first wood/coal getter, then Dennis and then me.

Our other chores consisted of caring for the huge garden. We had almost every vegetable one could think of; and Dad even made a fruit garden in our third year of being Elkhornites.

Hard work and bountiful harvests.

I remember the long hot summer days spent in the garden picking weeds, dusting the potatoes with powder to deter potato beetles and hilling the potato plants. Fall was an exciting time but it involved a lot of hard work. We had potatoes to dig and bag, corn to harvest and shuck, turnips, beets, carrots and so many more root vegetables that we picked and prepared to be stored in sand filled bins in the cellar. We often had corn roasts at this time and invited town folk enjoy some corn and help themselves to the excess of vegetables that were still left in the garden.

Mom canned pickles, beets, tomatoes, beans and so much more; enough to last until the next year's harvest. Yes, it was a lot of hard work but I believe it taught us the value of hard work, team work and being neighborly while providing us with good, fresh, healthy food.

The Trials and Tribulations of Gluten Free Baking.

Mom also worked hard but disappointingly to bake gluten free food for Elaine and me. Mom liked to bake and was an exceptionally good baker. She baked bread, pies, cookies and all kinds of "delicious goodies" twice a week. Mom was also a superb cook and cooked mostly British style; that is roast beef with Yorkshire pudding, stews with dumplings, meat pies, fish and chips, (battered) toast, hot cereals such as Red River Cereal and so on. Because Elaine and I could no longer eat any of Moms' baking; and many of the meals had to be altered to eliminate all the "good stuff".

In the mid-fifties and right up to the mid-eighties, there was no gluten free food to be found on the store shelves in a small rural town, not even in the cities. The only gluten free baking ingredient I recollect Mom having was corn flour and corn meal. Mom attempted to make bread using corn flour but of course, without gluten, it crumbled when one tried to make a sandwich with it. It did make a tasty desert when caramel sauce was poured over it!

I would also like to note that even though Elaine and I avoided the foods that were known to contain gluten, chocolate or fats, we were still unknowingly exposed to unknown sources of gluten in many other food products. These sources included but were not limited to foods such as oatmeal, malt flavored foods, hydrolyzed plant protein. We didn't have the convenient Pocket Dictionary - Acceptability of Foods & Food Ingredients for the Gluten-Free Diet produced and distributed by the Canadian Celiac Association which was started in 1972.

Another New Beginning, Time to Start School

As our first summer in Elkhorn drifted into fall, it was time to for me start school. This was my first year of school. It was for the most part uneventful and at the end of the year I was promoted to grade two.

In grade two my marks were Bs, Cs and Ds in the beginning of the year but ended with an A average and was promoted to grade three with honors.

As I continued through to grade eight I had increasing difficulty with mathematics. I always had low marks in math and from grade five on I consistently failed math. In grade seven, my teacher, Ms.

McCauley, recognized my weakness in math and kept me after school to help me with mathematics. As a result I achieved a grade of 79 in math and was promoted to grade eight. I passed grade eight with average grades and was promoted to grade nine.

Banana Buggy

I loved to tinker and build stuff. Our 'back shed' had a work bench and Dad kept his tools there. I asked Dad if I could use his tools to build a car. Dad was somewhat taken aback and repeated, "Build a car?" I said, "Yes, I want to build a soap box car." Dad replied with a glint in his eye, "You can use the tools but be careful and make sure you put them away when you're done and keep the shed clean." Yippy, I'm going to make the neatest car in town!

I started off with a 2 x 4 for the frame, then added 2 x 4's for the axel mounts. I nailed the rear axle mount to the 2 x 4 frame and had to find a bolt, 2 nuts and 4 flat washers to bolt the front axle mount centered on the 2 x 6. The wheels and axels were salvaged from an old baby carriage. Now I need some u nails to attach the axes to their mounts, but there were none available. I decided to put a few nails alongside the axel then bend them over to hold it in place.

Now I needed a piece of rope to tie to the steering axel so the driver could steer the car. I also needed some more wood to make a seat, seat back and a push stick. I jumped on my bike and rode to the hardware store and asked if they had any scrap wood I could have. They were always happy to oblige and showed me some broken pallets and scraps of wood and told me to help myself. I was able to find what I needed including some nylon twine which I took for the steering rope.

Back in the shed, the car was shaping up. I created a seat with a place for the push stick; made a push stick and installed the steering rope. The car was ready for a test run. I called Harvey and we met at the top of the hill near the school for the cars' inaugural test run.

After a few test runs I realized the axles were sliding back and forth along the mounts; and the steering was awkward, so, back to the drawing board we go. We also wanted to 'spice it up' with a steering wheel, front end, lights and so on.

First of all, we had to stop the axels from moving. I took them off and went to my Dad's shop to ask his advice. I thought I could drill two holes in each axel and screw it to the mount, then nail it as before.

Dad thought the idea of screwing the axels to their mounts was good. He went on to suggest making four blocks for each axel that would fit over the axel and attach to the mount using screws. This would keep the axel attached to the mount. I drilled the four holes in the axels and rode off back to the shed to rebuild our wheel mounting set-up.

One day when I went into Bartley's General Store through the back door, I noticed some tall, tapered baskets. When I went to the checkout counter, I asked if I could have one of the baskets. Don said, "They are banana baskets, I could have the broken one." So now we have a front end for our 'banana' car!

Over time and from here and there, Harvey and I found the various parts we needed to 'deck out our banana car'. Little by little it took shape until finally, we had a beautiful creation that included bicycle headlights, a horn, a steering wheel, hand brake and so much more!

Now onto High School

Grade nine was in the recently built high school, Elkhorn Collegiate Institute (ECI). I was anxious yet nervous about starting high school. As freshman, we were no longer the oldest group in the school, now we are the youngest. On the other hand, we are considered as young adults and are allowed more freedoms; but of course along with freedoms come consequences.

One of the differences from grade school to high school was that we had multiple teachers. This meant we had to learn what we could and couldn't get away with each teacher!

I recall on November 22, 1963, the day John F. Kennedy was assassinated, a classmate, Brian, returned from lunch ten minutes late. When Brian walked into the class room, our History teacher, Mr. M, demanded in a very loud voice, "Why are you late?" Brian replied that President Kennedy had been assassinated and he lost track of time while watching it on television. The whole class fell silent.

I was offered an after school job assisting the school custodian, Mr. McLeod. I worked every week day after class mopping floors throughout the school. When school breaks came, such as Christmas, we washed and waxed all the floors; and during summer break we washed all the walls, windows and floors then waxed and polished all the floors once again.

Eventually I was given the honor to raise the flag every morning; a task of which I took great pride in doing. One morning I raised the flag as usual and went to my class. Shortly thereafter, to my surprise, Mr. McLeod came to the classroom and asked to speak to me. Apparently the principal called him at home and complained the flag was upside down! I was so embarrassed! I apologized to Mr. McLeod and rushed out to upright the inverted flag. I never forgot that incident and was very alert from then on every time I raised that flag.

Now that I am a freshman, I was allowed to go to dances and other events around town. Quite often when we were out on the town, my buddies wanted to go for hamburgers, so, not wanting to be different, I would have a hamburger too. This happened quite frequently and in spite of having stomach cramps and diarrhea, I would still go for burgers.

Somehow, moms know everything and Mom knew I was getting into the forbidden foods; and given her frustration with trying to feed us, Mom loosened the reins on our diet, we were allowed a little bit of the gluten containing food from each meal. Of course, she did this not knowing the long term results of not adhering to the diet.

So life went on, I repeated grade nine. It was the Beatles fault and that's my story and I'm sticking to it! Then finally I was promoted to grade ten. It was 1965. The federal government established the Canada Pension Plan; Canada and the United States signed the Auto Pact in January; Canada inaugurated its new flag (red maple leaf on white with red side bars) on February 15; The Hydro-Electric Power Commission of Ontario inadvertently caused the great eastern seaboard blackout of '65 on November 9. Millions were left without electrical power for days and thousands were trapped in elevators until rescued. (Incidentally, a major baby-boom occurred 9 months later) and the Beatles' record-breaking first performance at New York's Shea Stadium was watched by 55,600 fans. They pocketed $160,000 of the $304,000 box office takings.

Finally, An Explanation For My Physical Limitations.

High schoolers are expected to perform in sports. At ECI, the important sports were basketball in the winter months, and track and field in the spring. Because of my height (6'-3" - 190.5 cm) I was expected to be a good player in basketball as well as track and field. I was asked to join the basketball team and was offered the position of Center. For whatever reason, I was very clumsy and did not do well in this position. I was then placed as Point Guard which involved less running and dribbling. I was better in this position as I was often able to block the opponent when trying to drop the ball through the basket.

Track and Field was another very disappointing trial for me. One of the challenges the coaches gave us was the four minute mile; my four minute mile was nine minutes at best! I was also considered a good candidate for High Jump and Hurdles. I also failed miserably at these two events in spite of trying very hard with hours of practice after school hours. I was embarrassed by a class mate who was much shorter than me yet able to high jump over six feet while my best was less than four feet.

In the winter many of my friends and classmates would skate in the rink or play street hockey. I had never tried skating so I obtained a pair of skates and went to the rink to learn how to skate. No matter what I did, I could not stand up on the skates; my feet would "flop over" at the ankle. After several weeks of trying, a friend, Ken F, said, "I have a pair of skates at home that might be better for you." We went to his house and got the skates and returned to the rink. The blade of the skate was not as high as regular skates and was much thicker. In researching images of the skates, they appear to be speed skates. I put them on and I was able to walk in them and when I hit the ice I could actually stay upright! So, thanks to Ken, I learned to skate (somewhat) and often joined in the street hockey games; usually as goalie because I was still much like a new born calf when I tried to maneuver the puck through and around moving targets! After participating in these street hockey sessions, I was very tired and cold. I would go home and sit as close as I could to the stove in the kitchen in attempt to warm up.

Another condition I experienced in my teens was numerous tooth aches. This occurred frequently but I didn't complain to my parents about them. When we were living in Winnipeg, we went to the dentist at least once a year. There was no dentist in Elkhorn so in my mind; there was no means of dealing with the issue, therefore no reason to tell Mom and Dad. One can be their own worst enemy at times!

At age forty eight I was diagnosed with peripheral neuropathy. When the doctor told me the diagnosis, I was of the belief that neuropathy was common for people with diabetes so I asked the doctor if I have diabetes. He explained that neuropathy can occur in people that do not have diabetes, and added that I was born with it. He then asked if I was active in sports and I told him of my struggles with skating and field day activities. He explained that the peripheral muscles are weakened by the nerve damage caused by neuropathy so now you know why you could not compete. In hearing this news I wanted to cry and laugh at the same time; finally an explanation for my physical limitations!

Peripheral neuropathy, a result of damage to your peripheral nerves, often causes weakness, numbness and pain, usually in your hands and feet. It can also affect other areas of your body.

Your peripheral nervous system sends information from your brain and spinal cord (central nervous system) to the rest of your body. Peripheral neuropathy can result from traumatic injuries, infections, metabolic problems, inherited causes and exposure to toxins. One of the most common causes is diabetes mellitus.

People with peripheral neuropathy generally describe the pain as stabbing or burning. Often, there's tingling. In many cases, symptoms improve, especially if caused by a treatable underlying condition. Medications can reduce the pain of peripheral neuropathy.

A recent study found that some people with celiac disease had neuropathic symptoms before the gastrointestinal symptoms of celiac disease appeared. The results of this study, and the fact that 10 percent of people with celiac disease suffer from an associated neurological condition (usually peripheral neuropathy or ataxia - a condition characterized by jerky, uncoordinated movements and gait), indicates that patients with neuropathy of an unknown cause should be tested for celiac disease. Adherence to a gluten-free diet lessens and/or eliminates almost all patients' symptoms.
By Mayo Clinic Staff

Imprudent decisions by a seventeen year old.

While in grade ten I thought I was doing well with my studies. I opted for business practice over French and I found the course quite interesting.

Mr. McLeod retired so I was no longer employed as custodial helper. After school I worked at my Dad's shop as I had done prior to working for Mr. McLeod. Dad taught me about working safely with the equipment and how to do a variety of jobs. He began teaching me to weld as well. In the winter time he teamed up with a welding supply dealer from Brandon to teach basic welding and sell home shop welding machines. I attended these classes as well if space permitted. When Dad felt I was capable, he would allow me to do some welding jobs. I enjoyed this type of work but never thought it would become my occupation, but it eventually did. I obtained journeyman steel fabricator certification as well as Canadian Welding Bureau certification and worked in the industry for twenty-seven years.

Back in grade ten, as many teenagers do, I was becoming impatient and wanting to become more independent. My Mom and I were not in accord on several topics; one being she did not want me to hang around with my best buddy, Harvey. She never explained why and I was quite frustrated. In March I rebelled and hitched a ride to Winnipeg with a local trucker; essentially quitting school just before final exams. I was seventeen and was determined to get a job and become my own boss. I arrived in Winnipeg and looked up Dennis who was living in a boarding house and working in a restaurant. I asked if I could stay with him until I could find a job. As Dennis always did, he supported me and advised me that I would likely not be able to obtain employment because I was still under eighteen and had no letter of authorization from Mom and Dad. Dennis was right, every business I approached asked my age, and did I have a letter of authorization from my parents or guardian. Dennis encouraged me to go back home and "stick it out", which I did.

So, just like the blockbuster fiasco, I had to face the wrath of Mon once again, only this time it was entirely my own doing! As it turned out, Mom and I never did discuss why she did not want me to hang out with Harvey; she had much bigger news to tell me. She told me, "Your Dad and I are putting the business and the house up for sale and we will be moving to Winnipeg in July".

I spent the rest of the school year helping at home and in the shop. I was told that, "If I return to school in Winnipeg they (Mom and Dad) would support me, but if I didn't return to school, I would have to get a job and support myself," meaning pay board and room if I stay at home. I decided to work for one year then get a part time evening job and go to Tech Voc High School to get my grade twelve and study Commercial Art.

CHAPTER FOUR

Back to Winnipeg

Getting settled in Winnipeg.

After eleven years in Elkhorn, we made the move again, in reverse. It was an emotional time for me, I grew up in Elkhorn, made some good friends and now we move to a city where I don't know anyone except Mom's siblings and their families. I did "re-connect" with my cousin Ray and to this day we are very good friends.

Mom asked Dennis to find a house for rent in Winnipeg which would be suitable for taking in boarders to supplement their income. Dennis found a well maintained house in the North Main area, close to bus service, grocery stores, etc.

I found employment and became a tenant in my parent's boarding house. For the two or three years that the boarding house existed, there was quite an interesting assortment of "characters" that came and went which kept life interesting and I imagine quite challenging for Mom. Tenants were provided with breakfast, lunch, (bag lunch on work days) and supper; the rooms were cleaned and bedding was washed every week.

Learning the ways of city life.

It wasn't long before I realized I was very conspicuous when I would board the transit bus in the morning to go to work. In Elkhorn it was customary to acknowledge everyone you met on the street, either with a "good morning" or a wave if in your vehicle; so as a green horn city slicker, I continued this tradition until I realized those vacant stares I was getting meant I must be doing something wrong. After some observation of people's behavior, I realized I was being perceived either as a "nut case" or a lost country boy. I eventually acclimatized to the way of city life I have become too accustomed to all the conveniences, and for that reason, although it's a pleasure to visit, I would not want to move back home to Elkhorn.

Derailed plans, employment and relationships.

Many things in my life occurred which derailed my plans to go to Tech Voc High School. At first, I tried two or three menial jobs but felt they were not suited for me; they were either too physically demanding or boring. I wanted to work at something I enjoyed. I responded to an ad for a "bell boy" position at the St. Regis Hotel and was hired. I enjoyed this position as I was able to interact with people and provide services to them.

During this time I experienced quite severe pain in my legs and back. There was a doctor's office across the street from the hotel so I went to see what was causing the pain. The doctor told me I had arthritis to which I retorted, "But I'm seventeen, aren't I too young to have arthritis?" The doctor explained that anyone of any age can develop arthritis.

It was at the St. Regis where I met Shirley, my future wife. After working at the St. Regis for about three years my relationship with Shirley was becoming more and more serious and marriage was looming, I decided to seek a more "responsible" line of work. As it happened, one of Mom's boarders was a postal worker and he told me how to apply for a job in the Post Office. I applied and was hired as a mail handler. A secure job with good benefits for life ... or so I thought!

I worked here for four years. During this time I was consistently being followed throughout the post office by a superintendent who was referred by the staff as "The Little General." This man was short on stature but had a thundering voice which he would use on occasion.

One benefit enjoyed by postal employees in the day was matrimonial leave. Employees who were getting married were given one week off with pay. On the occasion of my wedding, we planned to go to Ontario for the week and return home on Sunday evening as I was scheduled to return to work on the afternoon shift the following Monday.

A wedding, a hot car and chocolate milk.

Now that I have secure employment, I can ask Shirley to marry me. I went to Ben Moss and bought a ring with the assurance it could be exchanged. Then I proposed to Shirley that Christmas and she said, "Yes". After we returned to Ben Moss to exchange the ring for the one Shirley really, really wanted; we began making wedding plans. We didn't want a big, expensive wedding so planning was quite simple.

When we announced our engagement to our family's, Brother Dennis (now a chef and restaurant manager living in Carman, Manitoba) and his wife Donna, generously offered to make and host our wedding dinner.

We planned to have the wedding ceremony in Winnipeg and go out to Carmen for our wedding reception. Well, things didn't quite go as well as planned. Larry, a good friend from Elkhorn was my best man and he did a fantastic job. I worked the evening shift in the post office and invited my work mates over for a bit of a bachelor party. We got to my place about mid night and Larry had munchies, beer and assorted drinks all ready for us. We all sat around and shot the crap until about three AM.

The next morning, Larry and I had to decorate his brand new Ford car that he so graciously provided us for the wedding. We put the cake car topper on the roof; and it seemed like thousands of paper flowers all over the car. Finally, around noon, we finished the car and scrambled to get cleaned up and dressed for the wedding ceremony. Then we both rushed off; Larry in the wedding car to pick up Shirley and her aunt; and me in our Corvair to pick up my parents. Larry arrived at the church on time but I was a few minutes late but the ceremony went well thereafter.

Now it's time to head off to Carman. Shirley and I were in Larry's car sans the roof top cake decoration and my Dad drove the Corvair. We were still inside the Perimeter on McGillivray Blvd. when all of a sudden smoke began pouring out from under the hood of the Ford. Larry quickly pulled off to the shoulder and we frantically opened the hood to see a fire in the carburetor. We snuffed it out with an old blanket; then decided to push the car into the ditch for fear it may re-ignite and possibly explode. Luckily my parents showed up a few minutes later. After some discussion, Larry said he would have to go to the dealer so would not be able to attend the reception. We offered him a ride to the dealership and he replied, "You guys have a wedding reception to get to, I'll be okay". We objected but Larry won out and we went on our way in the Corvair.

We finally arrived at Dennis and Donna's, and when we entered their home, the smell of delicious food wafted throughout the house. They had a beautifully roasted turkey sitting proudly in the center of the table surrounded by dishes of potatoes, vegetables, gravy and salads; all in the style of a master chef!

We had a round of toasts and began the delicious celebratory dinner. We danced and partied until late in the evening, then we said our good byes and headed to the Corvair. The first thing I saw was a sign on the side of the car which read, "This isn't the Mayflower but many girls have come across in it, eh Ron!" I never thought about our car being "vandalized" but I guess it is all part of the celebrations. I got Shirley seated and went around to the driver's side. When I grabbed the steering wheel I got a hand full of goo! I immediately said, "Dennis, what did you do here?" Of course Dennis was in full denial as was everyone else. The goo leaked onto the seat cover; I removed the seat cover and wiped the goo off the steering wheel. There was also mud on the windshield so I turned on the wiper washer to clean the window and up came chocolate milk! As we attempted to leave the car wouldn't start. I made a lucky guess and checked the exhaust pipe for a blockage, and sure enough, there was a potato jammed into it! While I was back there, I also noticed "Just Married" written on the back of the car. Finally, we got on the road and first thing the next day we headed for a car wash before going on our honey moon.

We took full advantage of the matrimonial leave from the Post Office and honey mooned in Ontario. As luck would have it, on our way back home on Sunday, we were about two hundred miles from home when the Corvair began losing power. I didn't know what the problem was so I phoned my Uncle in Kenora, Ontario. He was an auto mechanic by trade and owned a marina in Kenora. I asked him if he would look at the Corvair; and to send a tow truck to bring the car to his shop. He sent the tow truck and when we arrived in Kenora, my uncle was not home. My aunt invited us to stay the night. In the morning, after my uncle examined the car and said, "The engine is shot." Given this news, I knew I would be not be able to get back to

Winnipeg in time for work so I phoned into work to explain my dilemma.

We caught a bus to Winnipeg and I returned to work the next afternoon. I had just started my shift when the Little General came over to my work area and bellowed, "Webster, get over here." I went over to him and he instructed me to follow him to the office. I didn't know what the issue was but I decided to take a union shop steward with me. I turned toward the shop steward and the Little General asked, "Where are you going?" I relied, "To get a union rep." He retorted, "You don't need a union rep." to which I responded, "It is my right to have a rep with me and I am not going into your office without one."

Upon entering the Little General's office, he began shouting "Why weren't you at work yesterday?" I explained my issues with the car and he kept 'grilling' me but did not ask for proof of my story. During this session, the Little General's boss (Mr. T) came by and when he heard the yelling, he came into the office and demanded an explanation for the shouting. The Little General stated. "Webster did not come to work yesterday." Mr. T asked me, "Is that true Ron?" to which I replied, "Yes." He then asked why and I told him of the issue with the car." He then asked, "Did you phone the H.R. Department to tell them you wouldn't be at work?" and again I replied, "Yes." He then asked if I have proof of the car being towed and that you took a bus home from Kenora. Upon producing a towing receipt and bust ticket receipts, Mr. T said, thank you, please return to your work stations. Upon closing the office door, we could hear more boisterous speaking, but this time from the mouth of a normally soft spoken Mr. T.

When Mr. T. retired, the Little General stepped up his observance of me, even to the degree of following me around the post office while I did my duties. For that reason after very much consideration, I decided no job was worth this kind of harassment, so I decided to go into the metal fabrication industry and use the skills my Dad taught me.

A family tragedy

Our one week honeymoon was over in a flash and it was time to go back to work and settle into married life.

One of Shirley's family's favorite things to do was camp and fish. My parents never camped or fished so this was a new adventure for me which I learned to enjoy. Overtime we bought a tent, camping equipment and camping became a summer weekend activity for us.

On one occasion in 1970, when we were on vacation, we stayed in a mobile at a campground in Petersfield, Manitoba. One day we got a surprise visit from my Aunt Aileen and Uncle Al who drove out to tell us my Mom was in the hospital and was not doing well. We quickly packed up and went back to Winnipeg; our first stop being the Health Science Center to visit Mom. Being unfamiliar with hospitals at the time, I was traumatized when I entered Mom's room, which I now believe was the Intensive Care Unit. Mom was not awake and had multiple tubes coming from her and machines beeping and blinking all around her. It has haunted me that I did not visit Mom in the hospital very often because it was such a traumatizing experience for me. Mom had lung cancer which was treated with surgery. Over the next eighteen months Mom courageously fought but it became evident she was losing the battle. On December 10th, 1971, Mom succumbed to the cancer in the Grace Hospital. Little did I know at the time this was the beginning of a way of life I would come to know all too well.

Christmas was a time for family and in spite of everyone's efforts to make it a happy occasion, it was quite somber. Mom was always the spark we all needed when it came time for family gatherings.

Time to visit a dentist

By now my dental situation was not good. There were more 'bad' teeth than good one so I decided to have them all extracted and get dentures. I attended three different dentist who all told me they would remove the decayed teeth but I still had six 'good' teeth. I asked the reasoning behind that and was told, "Those are the only teeth you will ever have so we should preserve as many as we can." Given that there were only six good teeth, I assumed the purpose for this was a means to make more money in the future, so I declined and they refused to extract all my teeth.

Later I learned of the dental students offering dental services as part of their training and went to consult with them. The Doctor in charge agreed to extract my teeth, two or three at a time, three times per week. This idea started off great but after each visit I required more and more local anesthetic and frequently the students would 'hit a nerve'. This 'unnerved' me and after having about twelve teeth extracted, I did not return.

Later, I was advised of a dentist that was quite well respected so I attended his office. I explained my plight and he replied, "I will extract the remainder of your teeth and give you a set of dentures. We will do this in the hospital where you will be more comfortable." It seemed my struggle was near an end.

On the day of the dental surgery, I went to the hospital and by four o'clock that afternoon; I went home with a brand new set of choppers! I was told to allow the gums to heal for several days and that my gums will shrink somewhat and I may have to have the dentures relined.

As it turned out, my gums shrunk more than expected and beyond the denturist's ability to make them fit. So I have just spent over $500 and still have no teeth. At various times I would go to a dentist to inquire about being fitted with dentures but they explained I would need bone surgery to enable them to fit properly. It wasn't until 2011 that I found a dentist who could provide me with dentures without having surgery.

Celiac attack

For the most part, up until now, I was functioning quite well. I had the usual bouts of diarrhea and ongoing dental problems but now

I am experiencing frequent chills that not even layers of comforters and heating pads could abet. On a few occasions Shirley called our family physician in the middle of the night. Dr. M. came to examine me but could find no cause for my chills.

After a few incidences of chills I began to think back to my childhood in the earlier days of the diagnosis of celiac. I could not recall the name (celiac disease) but I did remember the word gluten. I went to the library and requested information about gluten. My search turned up several books about celiac disease, a number of which I borrowed and read for clues of a relationship with celiac and my medical condition. Sure enough, some of the known symptoms of celiac disease included diarrhea, the chills (anemia) and a host of other maladies.

Upon learning this, I went to see Dr. M and told him about my diagnosis of celiac disease when I was a child. He immediately recognized the symptoms I was experiencing were likely related to celiac disease and that I should avoid gluten. Another bit of information I gained from the material obtained from the library was about the Canadian Celiac Association and that they had published the booklet "Acceptability of Food and Food Ingredients for the Gluten -Free Diet". I was informed that the Society of Manitobans with Disabilities have a library from which this booklet can be purchased. I obtained a copy and began a seemingly never ending marathon of reading labels as I shopped up and down the aisles of supermarkets.

Avoiding gluten was not so easy in the early seventies. I personally am not aware of any available gluten free food products in Winnipeg until about the mid-1980s. I recall hearing that Meyer's Drug Store on William and Salter had some gluten free products. I rushed to the store and was extremely happy to find gluten free bread, pastas from Europe and some macaroon cookies. I bought a loaf of frozen rice bread, a package of two macaroon cookies and a small package of pasta. The bread was about $5, the cookies were 99¢ and the pasta was over $7 for about 12 ounces. Obviously the cost of gluten free food was prohibitive but it was a start which brought hope for the future.

For those who have not experienced the "early" days of commercially available gluten free food, I can tell you we are very fortunate to have the glut and quality of gluten free food that is currently available. The frozen rice bread was a blessing in its time but it was a challenge in comparison to today's soft breads. At best, it needed to be toasted in order to make a sandwich that would not shatter at first bite! The pasta was a treat and indistinguishable from wheat based pasta but very costly. Today's prices for gluten free food are still significantly higher than "normal" food but in comparison to the earlier products, the price has been lowered substantially.

As time went on, little by little, gluten free foods began to appear in supermarkets. Safeway began selling the frozen brick of rice bread, and to my surprise one day as I was "on the hunt" I found some Mrs. Leepers gluten free corn pasta (elbows and spaghetti). It was about double the cost of wheat based pasta products but much cheaper than the pastas from Europe. So now we have a source of bread and pasta! Spaghetti and meatballs in tomato sauce were on the menu that night!

CHAPTER FIVE

Medical Issues

In the early 1980s I was happily employed designing and fabricating weldment jigs and fixtures. This job was challenging and I enjoyed every day of it. I had always had some back issues and had consulted my family physician about it He determined it was osteoarthritis and prescribed Voltaren™ which was significantly effective. One morning as I was getting out of bed I fell to the floor. My low back was in severe pain and I could not stand. I phoned my employer to notify them I would not be going to work, and then called my doctor. I explained that I could not walk and was unable to come to his office. He came to see me that evening. I was instructed to sleep on the floor until I was mobile again, and then make an appointment to see him. I was referred to an orthopedic surgeon who explained to me that I have osteoarthritis in my spine as well as degenerative disc disease. In viewing the x-rays of my low back, the deteriorated discs were quite evident. Three vertebrae were sitting bone on bone. The reason I could not walk is that the nerves going into my legs were pinched causing meralgia paresthesia.

Arthritis, Inflammation Cause Joint Pain

When your joints hurt, it could be due to arthritis, which involves the breakdown of cartilage in the joints themselves. It also could be due to inflammation of muscles and cartilage that make up that joint. Joint pain occurs more frequently as you get older, especially if you're overweight.

However, it's not entirely clear what triggers the joint pain in people with celiac disease. The pain occurs in people of every age, including children, and frequently waxes and wanes, depending on gluten ingestion.

Since the intestinal damage in celiac causes malnutrition, the pain could stem from nutritional deficiencies.

It also could stem from overall inflammation provoked by gluten ingestion, which could be what's happening in gluten sensitivity.

www.abouthealth.com

The orthopedic surgeon advised that I change into a different line of work as steel fabrication and welding was too strenuous for me. At the time I was designing and building weldment jigs and fixtures; and later I became involved in research and development which was 70% design work and 30% testing so there was much less physical stress. I did take the advice seriously and attended evening classes at Red River Community College.

For the next 2 plus years I was kept extremely busy juggling a full time job, drafting studies and my home life. After finishing my fourth term I was exhausted so took one term off. I returned for the winter semester and finally obtained certification in Advanced Level Machine Drafting and Engineering Design.

My employer offered me a position in the engineering department but at half the salary I was making. In retrospect, I should have accepted but did not, thinking only of the immediate situation. My thoughts on this now are, "If I worked so hard to learn drafting, I could have found part time work to supplement my income until I became more experienced in drafting, thus be paid more" ...but it wasn't my first stupid decision, nor will it likely be my last!

Then the unthinkable occurred, the company I was working for, the one I thought was going to last me for my working life, closed, went out of business! I was quite devastated. In spite of my training and experience in the industry, I was unable to find drafting/design work because now they are using computers and I had no experience with computers. I found other employment in which my certification in fabrication and welding, as well as layout and drafting skills were a prominent factor in obtaining this employment. This allowed me to continue working more in the design/layout aspect of projects rather than the heavier work of fabrication and welding.

It felt like a death sentence.

In 1993 I was diagnosed with testicular cancer. I was devastated. My thoughts went to my memories of how Mom suffered for so long, thinking I will have the same fate. As the saying goes, I began "putting my affairs in order."

I had surgery and then was referred to Cancer Care Manitoba. On my first visit, as I walked down the hall towards my oncologist's office, there were several young children playing and walking around, all had catheters of various types, many with no hair. They were cancer patients and were receiving chemotherapy. My immediate thoughts were, "Why am I so devastated? At least I've had a life; these little tykes haven't even begun their life yet, and maybe never will". I have never forgotten the sight I saw that day, and when things get a little tense for me, my mind goes back to that day and I immediately "suck it up". I also frequently think of my hero, Terry Fox, Terry gives me inspiration to keep up the fight without self-pity.

I completed radiation therapy that summer and returned to work in the fall.

Two years later I experienced Déjà vu. I now have cancer in the right testicle. On this occasion, I had surgery and was followed by oncologists at the St. Boniface Hospital. I would go twice per month for blood tests, x-rays, CT Scans and physicals. There were no signs of cancer after two years so I was advised that I would no longer require follow up by the oncologists, but maintain regular contact with my family physician.

Family strife.

Things at home have not been going so well. Shirley was very unhappy; I suppose partly because of the cancer and the resulting consequences. After thirty years of marriage with the last 8 or more years of our relationship deteriorating, I felt it was at the point of no return and made the decision to separate.

One other disappointment in our married life was our inability to have children. I do accept responsibility for not seeing our physician to determine if it was my lack of sperm or ... I now know celiac often is a cause of gonadal dysfunction.

A study from the Department of Medicine at Tampere University Hospital and Medical School at the University of Tampere Finland found that the rate of celiac disease among women reporting infertility was 4.1%. Although the exact reason for the increased risk remains unknown, the researchers suggested that female celiac patients who are not adhering to a gluten-free diet have a shortened reproductive period and early menopause. Males with celiac disease have shown gonadal dysfunction, which could also contribute to fertility complications.

The National Foundation for Celiac Awareness

I rented an apartment with occupation for January 2000 and moved on the first of January. After a few months we had several discussions on the phone and we met two times thereafter but reconciliation was not to be.

Moving on ...

Soon after settling in, I decided to combine my love of art and woodworking and create wooden signs. I purchased some wood working equipment and designed signs and patterns on the computer. I very much enjoyed doing this and made several signs for family members; then I began getting requests from people who had seen my signs so it became a hobby business. Eventually I began going to craft shows and displaying my products in craft shops. I began getting quite a few orders and decided to try designing other products such as desk clocks, fun signs, etc. One product I designed and became quite popular was a sign with the words, "We Don't Dial 911" and a rifle suspended below the sign board.

This is getting serious!

As time went on I kept quite busy but I began feeling ill. I was very tired and became quite weak. I went to my family physician but no diagnosis. I continued to go to various clinics and was frequently told to use laxatives as I was "constipated". This went on for several months until I went back to my family doctor. This time I was scheduled for a CT scan.

At Christmas time (2001) I was invited to attend the "Christmas Craft Show" at the (Hudson) Bay Downtown store. I had a display of my products in the craft section (basement) and was given an opportunity to promote my products. I attended on two Saturdays; on the second Saturday I began feeling unwell and had to leave.

On the 29th of December, I awoke and barely had the energy to get out of bed. I called my sister, Elaine, and asked her if she would take me to the E.R. at St. Boniface Hospital. Little did I know, my life was about to change in a very radical way.

We arrived about 10:00 a.m. and were taken into the emergency room after a short wait. That's when the day became very long. I waited for two or three hours in the examining room when finally a doctor came to ask why I was there. I explained how I was feeling, that I was unable to eat and hadn't had a bowl movement for quite some time. He poked and prodded me and said he was going to send his colleague in to see me. After some time, another doctor appeared and asked questions and prodded me and said, "We don't see anything serious going on with you so we are going to send you home." I retorted that, "If I die the onus will be on you." He was quite taken aback and asked, "Do you really think there is something that serious going on with you?" I repeated what I had already stated to him and to the previous doctor; I had no other description for what I was feeling or experiencing. Since I had been to so many doctors and clinics and my condition continues to worsen, I believed I required immediate medical attention. The doctor said, "We will get some blood work done and go from there."

After a fairly long wait, the doctor returned and stated, "The blood work indicated I was anemic and there was another concern they had and I would be getting an x-ray." By the time I went for an x-ray it was getting late in the day. Finally another doctor came in to tell me, "They do see something in the x-ray but it is unclear so I will order a C.T. scan."

It was about 10:30 p.m. when they wheeled me out of the C.T. scan room. I was not returned to the E.R. I don't know where I was but the doctor came over to me and said he needed to confer with another doctor. He went to a nearby phone then returned stating, "We are going to admit you for further observation."

Sunday was a quiet day but on Monday Doctor D, a surgeon came to see me and explained he I have colon cancer and require surgery. Then I was given an enema and two nurses attempted to install a nasogastric tube but I was choking and gagging and it seemed there was just no way was it going to happen. One of the nurses said, "This tube will be inserted, even if we have to do it when you are in surgery."…and that's when it was inserted.

People with celiac disease who don't maintain a gluten-free diet have a greater risk of developing several forms of cancer, including intestinal lymphoma and small bowel cancer.

Mayo Clinic

Surgery was slated for Tuesday January 2nd (2001) but after waiting until about 4 p.m., Doctor D. came into my room and said, "I am so sorry, I will not be doing your surgery today because I have been in surgery all day and am very tired. I do not want to operate when I feel like this. I will reschedule your surgery to 9:00 a.m. tomorrow morning." I appreciated Dr. D's honesty which bumped him up a notch on my confidence scale.

The surgery happened as scheduled and my first memory when waking was seeing my brother Ken and his wife Gail in the post op room. They were a welcome sight but I wonder to this day how they were able to visit me in post op.

Eventually I was moved to a ward and began my recovery. I was feeling very weak and of course unable to eat with the nasogastric tube inserted. As time went on my condition did not seem to be improving. A night nurse quietly checked on me several times throughout the night. One night she woke me up with a loud, "Yahoo!" She was holding up my pouch of urine and said, "Look at this"! I didn't know what to say, then she added, "The colour is perfect, you are starting to recover!"

On Friday afternoon, (January 11th) the doctor replacing Doctor D. (who was on holidays), walked through the ward and pointed at me and said, "You're going home tomorrow." My nurse objected loudly saying, "He has not even been able to eat yet, we don't even know if he can tolerate food!" The doctor then said, "We'll keep you until Sunday then, you had best start eating." Needless to say, I was not impressed by his haughty attitude and lack of compassion,

Sunday came along and out of the hospital I went. I was given instructions to see Dr. D. in two weeks. I was very weak, could not walk and had only some fluids since the surgery. I knew I was being discharged much too early but I had no say in the matter. I stayed with Elaine and her family until February 2nd. I was still quite weak and had not been able to eat very much as yet. Upon returning home, within a few days I began gaining strength and my appetite improved immensely. I guess the old saying; "There is no place like home," is true.

A Change of Direction

By May I was still quite weak and found that I could not continue my hobby business at a sustainable level. I was very disappointed as I enjoyed doing the work. During my recovery from surgery I read a lot of magazines. One magazine had an ad which was offering a book on how to create portrait patterns from photographs and cut them out using a scroll saw thus creating "wooden portraits". I was very intrigued by this concept and ordered the book. After a few weeks of practice on the computer I began creating patterns that were acceptable. I joined an online self-help group which was formed by the author of the book and whose membership was other scrollers who were interested in either making patterns or creating wooden portraits.

Eventually my ability to create patterns from photos became well known and I decided to pursue this as a hobby business. I could do business online which meant much less physical effort and I could work on my own schedule.

I acquired help to build a website and after a few trials and tribulations my business became profitable with minimal overhead. I not only created patterns from photos but also of the "things of life". The patterns I most enjoyed creating most were classic cars, and they were immensely popular. Other patterns included celebrities and TV /movie stars, landscapes, dogs, cats, wild animals and desk toppers.

Some of the most memorable patterns were one I did of Loretta Lynn for a client who was a friend of Loretta's. The photo was of Loretta standing in front of her newest tour bus with the banner "Coal Miner's Daughter" across the front. This portrait is proudly displayed in Loretta's Museum on her ranch in Hurricane Mills, Tennessee. Another one was of Meryl Haggard; a devout fan had front row tickets to Meryl's concert and wanted to give him a portrait and have him sign a second one. Apparently Meryl was quite impressed with the portrait and autographed the copy.

I operated this business until 2012 when I realized the popularity of it was dwindling and it was no longer profitable.

More Health Concerns

As time went on, un-noticed by me, I was gaining weight. I attended my family doctor every four months and he brought it to my attention that I had gained a lot of weight and must go on a diet. I explained that, I was fearful of not eating enough and would end up back in the hospital. I added, I was told by the nurses at the Grace to keep my potassium level up (salt and bananas). He suggested cutting back on the salt and going to 'Weight Watcher's. I requested a dietician because 'Weight Watchers' had no gluten free options. I attended a dietician and was given some very good advice. I was in the habit of skipping breakfast and had no set time for meals. I was informed that our body requires consistent eating habits, and that breakfast is the most important meal of the day. I began trying to eat more consistently and over time I ate three meals a day at specific times.

I had become much less active due to a lower energy level and because I was doing more work on the computer making patterns instead of shop work and traveling to craft vendors and shows.

At some point in time I decided a mobility scooter would prove useful, especially for getting groceries. I did research on the internet to learn what was available and at what cost. I realized I could not afford a new one so began looking for used ones.

One did catch my eye, the price seemed right and recently had new batteries installed. The phone number to contact the seller seemed familiar but I could not place it until good my friend Randy answered the phone. I asked, "Is this Randy?" to which he answered, "Non other!" I told him why I was calling and that I had a senior moment about his phone number.

The next day Randy brought the scooter over and although it appeared in very good condition, it required new rear tires. I felt that wasn't a deal breaker so we made the deal.

I called mobility scooter company a few blocks away from my apartment and asked him about tires and if he would check over the scooter and report it's condition to me. He asked me about batteries and I told him they were replaced six months ago. Leo soon arrived to pick up the scooter and took it back to his shop. Soon afterward, he called and asked me again about the batteries. I told him I just bought the scooter and the seller told me they were replaced six months ago. Leo said, "These batteries are not new, one is three years old, the other four years old and they are two different brands." Having been the victim of a scam or two, I thought maybe Leo wanted to sell me batteries as well as tires. I asked him, "Are you sure of this?" He replied, "Yes I am sure, you must have been scammed by the seller." I informed him that, "I bought the scooter from a friend whom I've known since 1975 and who has never cheated me or misrepresented himself in any way. I trust my friend." Leo replied, "I have two customers here right now, I suggest you come over and look for yourself. I am not about to scam you or anyone else, I was an

R.C.M.P. Officer for twenty-five years and worked in security for twenty years, so I have two good pensions." I told Leo I would call Randy and get back to him."

I called Randy at work, told him what Leo said, and asked him about the batteries. Randy said "I took the scooter to the battery place and left it with them; they phoned when it was ready and I went to pick it up without checking the batteries. Randy then retrieved the invoice for the batteries which had no serial numbers or other identifying information. Randy called the owner of the battery shop and within two hours, two new batteries were delivered to Leo's shop and I called to apologize that I doubted him.

As it turned out, the scooter was below capacity for me (something I never considered when buying it) so I was on the hunt for a bigger one. Leo obtained a used 350 pound capacity scooter with twelve inch wheels, it was like a Cadillac and we were able to strike a deal. Now I have regained some of my independence!

An Interesting Project

Randy and I frequently collaborate on a variety of projects, mostly mechanical or structural. This time we got involved in the design and fabrication of a parallel arm tracer/carving machine. Randy's nephew, Aaron was from a musical family; his grandfather had a band for years; his father was an accomplished musician as was his older brother, Andrew. Aaron was also able to play several instruments but his desire was to build guitars and in doing so would require a machine that could shape and carve in 3D. Since I had been in the business of designing and building machines, Randy asked me to come in on this project. The machine was designed to trace an outline or profile of an object and cut it out or carve the profile with a router; as required for solid wood electric guitar bodies. Aaron's budget was quite small as he was attending university. We scrounged for materials and obtained the best parts we could within the budget and went to work. The machine was to be attached to a flat surface using rails and lineal bearings. The parallel arms were fabricated from metal and were attached to the lineal bearings in a manner that allowed the tracing and carving heads to pivot and swing almost 180 degrees. We had the machine assembled to the point of fabricating mountings for the tracer and router when I began feeling ill. The next thing I knew, I was back in the hospital

CHAPTER SIX

The Fight of my Life

It was 2007; Elkhorn's 125th Homecoming, and it promised to be a big event with a multitude of people expected to come back home. Elaine, Dennis and I made plans a year in advance and we were all excited about "going back home" in August to reunite with good friends and old acquaintances.

In April, I experienced very similar issues to that of my colon cancer in 2000-2001. I immediately knew that I had colon cancer again and decided I would not to seek medical intervention. Elaine phoned me as my condition was worsening and she recognized I was ill. She asked what was wrong and I said I just have the flu. She replied, "It sounds worse than just the flu, you should go to the hospital." I said, "I will be alright", and Elaine replied, "I am coming to take you to the hospital."

Elaine arrived in about half an hour, I relented and Elaine took me to the Grace Hospital which was only two blocks from my apartment on Country Club Boulevard. It was about 9:30 or 10:00 p.m. when we arrived at the Grace. I was triaged and admitted shortly thereafter.

When the doctor arrived he asked why I came to the E.R. I replied, "I have colon cancer." He was somewhat disconcerted and asked, "How do you know you have colon cancer?" I said, "I had it six years ago and I am experiencing the very same symptoms as I was then." He said, "Let's hope you are wrong." and sent me for an x-ray. The x-ray showed something unusual but indistinguishable and I was sent for a C.T. Scan. Immediately after the C.T. scan I was admitted into the hospital.

It was déjà vu; the nasogastric tube was inserted (this time prior to going into surgery), they gave me an enema and the next day off to surgery I go. A few hours later I'm back in my room and everything seemed to be as expected. After a few days the nasogastric tube was taken out (what a relief). Now it's time to restart my digestive system with some clear fluids. I was given some broth, jello and tea. I had a little of the broth and jello, but within a few minutes it came back up. This went on repeatedly over the next few months and the nasogastric tube had to be reinserted each time. Eventually, the tube was just pinched off when I was allowed to retry fluids.

On May 1st Dennis was in the Grace Hospital's Day Surgery unit. He was scheduled for hernia repair surgery. It was Dennis' 63rd birthday. The nurse asked Dennis, "What is your birth date?" Dennis replied, "May 1, 1944." The nurse said, "Yes, today is May 1, but I want you to tell me your birth date." This was repeated two or three times then the nurse said, "Oh my, are you telling me it is your birthday today?" Dennis replied, "Yes, and I expect a big birthday cake when I get back from surgery!" Of course the cake never materialized, but Dennis endured the surgery quite well.

After his surgery, Dennis was visited by Major Gordon (Salvation Army Chaplain). During their conversation Dennis told Gordon his brother Ron was on the fourth floor recovering from surgery. He asked Gordon to deliver the message to me that he is doing fine, and to come back to tell him how I am doing. So that is my first of many meetings with Gordon. Gordon has since retired and we still keep in touch and meet for coffee on occasion. On Dennis' passing in 2013, the family asked Gordon to officiate at Dennis' Celebration of Life. I have also requested that he preside over my memorial.

Dr. DI came to see me frequently and would pace back and forth at the foot of my bed. He was very caring and concerned and tried numerous methods of trying to determine why I was unable to retain food. I recall one attempt was to have a series of x-rays taken over one hour intervals. The purpose of this was to follow some dye that I was given through my digestive system in search for a blockage or other possible reason for my condition. This test began at 9 a.m. and continued until 10 p.m. and again the next day from 9 a.m. until about 2 p.m. In spite of multiple images per session, there were no definitive conclusions drawn from all the x-rays.

By July, after numerous attempts to feed me, I requested to be discharged citing that I believed it was the hospital food that turned me off. Dr. DI didn't agree with me that it was the hospital food, but at this point he was willing to try almost anything. Of course it wasn't the hospital food; I still wasn't able to eat. During this time I was prepped for chemotherapy. I went into the oncology clinic at the Grace for my first dose of chemo and was fitted with a chemo pump, I then returned two days later to have the pump removed. I returned to

Elaine and Leo's home where I was staying and crashed on my bed. I slept for four hours and when I woke up I was very hungry. Elaine made some bacon and eggs for me, and I had two helpings! My appetite was short lived and within a week I was back in the hospital. Now I had severe diarrhea and I lost almost all my hair.

I remained in the emergency department for five nights. After the second night I asked, "Why am I not being admitted?" I was told that Dr. H has to be the one to admit me but she hasn't been to the E.R. yet. I asked if she was aware of me being there and they said certainly, she was notified the minute you came into the E.R. Dr. H showed up on the fifth day and I was finally admitted, but to the fifth floor. The hospital is divided into sections of different types of services. For example, the Grace's fourth floor south is dedicated to surgery patients. No one would tell me what specialty the fifth floor offered but I soon realized that it is the floor where terminal patients are housed. Wow, why doesn't someone tell me my life is over!

Over the next two months, my oncologist (Dr. H.) visited me two or three times a week and each time she would ask, "Why are you in bed, you should be up walking!". Each time I replied, "I have a physiotherapist and I exercise and walk with her three times a day." On one occasion she came into my room when Elaine was visiting. An LPN followed her into the room to listen to what she had to say. Dr. H proceeded to tell me that there is nothing anyone could do for me. She said, "We will put you into palliative care." I replied, "Are you telling me I'm dying?" She replied, "No, palliative care doesn't mean you are dying, they take very good care of you there." She had us all in tears then left. Finally one day when Dr. H. came into my room and demanded I get out of bed. I asked her, "As an oncologist, can you do anything for me?" She replied, "No, there is nothing anyone can do for you." I politely asked her to just leave me alone. She made an abrupt exit and never returned.

Palliative care is an approach to care which focuses on comfort and quality of life for those affected by life-threatening illness. Its goal is much more than comfort in dying; palliative care is about living, through meticulous attention to control of pain and other symptoms, supporting emotional, spiritual and cultural needs and maximizing functional status. Palliative care is not a physical location but a philosophy of care at the end-of-life.

The WRHA Palliative Care Program provides services for people in Winnipeg who have been diagnosed with a life-limiting illness. The Palliative Care Program is based on the belief that quality end-of-life care can be provided in a variety of settings, with the preferred location of care being the home or other usual residence (such as a personal care home). Palliative Care Program resources and services support and enhance the ability of the patient's primary care team to continue to care for them at the end-of-life. Specialized units exist for patients whose needs cannot be met in other settings.

Winnipeg Regional Health Authority

I was severely depressed by this time and I felt that if I could not live, then I wanted to die. Thankfully my friend Major Gordon visited me frequently. We talked about life and prayed together. It is because of Gordon's frequent visits and his heartfelt caring, as well as Elaine's, Dennis' and friend Randy's support that I was eventually able to overcome the depression.

As time went on my life remained in limbo. One night I was extremely restless and kept getting out of my bed and back in again. I began to think I was losing my mind. I didn't know why I was doing what I was doing. Finally, about 6 a.m., I fell asleep. At about 7 a.m. a nurse woke me and she asked if I was feeling well. I replied, "I wasn't able to sleep all night and now I'm tired." She rushed away and I went back to sleep. Suddenly I awoke and there were nurses all around me and Dr. DI was standing at the foot of the bed. Dr. DI asked, "Are you not feeling well Ron?" I repeated that, "I had not slept during the night and was just feeling tired." Elaine called my extension and when I answered she asked, "Are you alright?" She added, "Dr. DI called and left a message that I had taken a turn for the worse and that the family should come to the hospital." Again I repeated that, "I had not slept during the night and was just feeling tired."

I was moved to an observation room and Dr. DI came by about every hour. Later in the day I was sent for a C.T. scan and after the scan I looked up there was Dr. DI. I asked him, "Is there something seriously wrong Dr. DI?" to which he replied, "No, I just wanted to get the results of this scan." Finally, on the third day, Dr. DI came to see me and said, "I'm happy to see you are looking better Ron, you had a 'bug in your blood' and we almost lost you. We gave you antibiotics but they didn't work so we tried a stronger antibiotic."

More Surgery.

More time passes with no changes other than it was determined that I required to be feed intravenously because my body was deteriorating. They were not the tastiest meals I've ever had but they did the trick.

I believe it was late September when Dr. DI came to visit me and he appeared to be preoccupied. He paced back and forth as he often did, then turned to me and said, "Ron, I think I can get you back home to live a relatively normal life, but it involves more surgery." I replied, I'm game for anything at this time, I have nothing to lose." He asked, "Do you know what a colostomy is?" I replied, "I have heard of them but virtually know nothing about them." Dr. DI went on to explain, "I believe the reason you cannot eat is because, during the surgery to remove the tumor from your colon, the nerves did not reconnect between the small colon and the large colon. A colostomy will enable us to bypass the large bowl and your waste will go into a pouch which will be attached to your abdomen. You will be trained by an Ostomy Nurse on how to maintain the pouch." Since it was the only hope I had been given in the past 5 months, I fully agreed to it. He said, "I will schedule the O.R. for the earliest date I can get". The next day Dr. DI came back. He appeared quite dejected. He said, "The earliest I can schedule the O. R. is in the new year." I was very disappointed. It looked like I would be spending Christmas with all my doctors, nurses and health care friends. Nice people, but not family!

The very next day, Dr. DI came into my room; he seemed quite invigorated and said, "Ron, I will be in the O. R., not this weekend, next weekend, doing emergency surgery. I will put you on my roster but you have to understand, all emergency cases come before you. If I get a chance I will bring you in for your surgery either on Saturday or Sunday. "My hopes were renewed; perhaps I will be home for Christmas with my family!

Well, the big day came; I was wide awake at 7 a.m. and by 9 a.m. I was all ready for surgery. The day dragged on and on, at about 3:30 I realized it's unlikely to happen today and put my hopes on Sunday.

Sunday morning came and, just like Saturday, I was ready and willing to go, but again, by 3:30 my hopes began to dwindle. Then suddenly, around 4 p.m., two attendants arrived and announced, "It's your turn!" I was finally being wheeled down for surgery!

I woke up in post op sometime around 8 p.m. I was quite surprised the surgery took that long. I could see a stream of people leaving, and then a very tired looking Dr. DI appeared in the post op unit. I thanked him for getting me in and working so late (he began surgery at 7 a.m. that day). As Dr. DI is, he would not take full credit for it. He replied, "It's not just me, it was all those people who are just leaving too."

I was placed in a room on the third floor to recover. On the third day after surgery, my nasogastric tube was pinched off and I was given clear fluids. Everything went well and on the next day I was given real food. I ate most of the tray contents and prepared to be sick, but it never happened! I am elated! I developed quite an appetite and began feeling better every day.

On the fourth day I woke up to a blood soaked bed. I could not see where the blood was coming from so I called the nurse. Apparently my incision had opened up. She immediately called the surgeon on duty then began "packing "the wound. The surgeon appeared and advised that they use negative-pressure wound therapy, (NPWT). I was returned to the fourth floor south, surgery ward where the NPWT machine was attached. This method would apparently close the incision without stiches and would heal within ten days.

The NPWT machine was installed and I felt like an eviscerated turkey covered in shrink wrap! I was quite active by now and in order for me to walk I had to load up the NPWV machine onto a walker. It was a bit bulky but not overly heavy. I did this for about ten or twelve days then the machine was removed. The NPWV could not close the whole wound, about on inch remained open and had to be attended to on a daily basis.

More Setbacks

Now my being discharged was the topic du jour. My open incision would require a nurse to come to my home and I would require home care. As each day went by, I was more and more active and my appetite was very healthy. I always looked forward to breakfast as each one was different and included gluten free cereal;

and on occasion a muffin or toast. I was still turned off by the hospital food; in particular, lunch and supper. Because of my gluten free requirement, both meals were potatoes, meat or fish and vegetables. The taste of these dishes was indistinguishable from one another. I asked Elaine to bring some food so that I could substitute the lunches and suppers, Elaine brought up several different meals which were kept in the staff's fridge. At meal time I would go to the staff room to get my lunch or supper and heat it up in the microwave

I felt ready to be discharged but there was a glitch in getting my home care organized. I remained in the hospital for another three weeks, and then finally I was informed that I will be going home the next day. The next day came and there was yet another hold up in my discharge. I was told I would be discharged in the evening. In spite of this, things worked out for the better. My cousin Lynda and her husband Wilf were in town and came to visit me. Since I was mobile and Elaine was waiting with me for my discharge, we decided to meet in the cafeteria. We took a wheel chair just in case I couldn't walk there and back. I was able to walk without becoming too tired so I suggested Elaine get into the wheel chair and go for a ride. As I pushed Elaine into the cafeteria Lynda stood up with a very "confused" look on her face! Elaine stood up and walked to the table as everyone remarked, "Now that's a different picture."

At about 7:30 word came that I am free to go. I had mixed feelings, I was very happy to finally be able to go home after seven long months in the hospital; but also a fear of experiencing further complications and having to return to the Grace. Luckily, I was able to return to a "modified" normal life as I learned to live with my new "Buddy" (Ileostomy).

Home Care informed me that I would have someone come in the morning to make breakfast, and then on Mondays and Thursdays they would return to aid me in having a shower. Another worker would come on Tuesdays and Thursdays to pre-make lunches and suppers and clean the apartment and do laundry. That's a lot of help, and traffic!

Christmas 2007

Our family tradition was that each of our sibling's families would take turns hosting Christmas dinner. This year was hosted by Dennis and his partner Ken. As usual, everyone brought their signature dish and we all had a delicious Christmas dinner together. This year was quite different for me; not only do I have to be on the lookout for gluten containing foods, now I have to be aware of foods that my new "Buddy" will object to. These foods include gaseous foods or foods that may cause blockages. When it came to Gail's Holopchi, I took a helping of filling along with a three inch square of cabbage, thinking "one little piece isn't going to be a problem". By evenings end, I thought I had managed to make the right selections and did not expect any issues. Well, I was wrong, one little piece of cabbage can and did cause a big problem! About 3 a.m. I awoke to find my Buddy had 'exploded'! I feel neither the desire nor need to explain this further!

Learning to Live With "Buddy"

The Christmas cabbage calamity was an eye opener as to how sensitive ileostomies could be. Along with the information provided me by the Enterostomal Therapy (E.T.) Nurses, I searched the internet for information from other sources. The following information describes day to day life for an ostomate. Please note: if you are squeamish about such topics, you may find some of this information gross, disgusting or down right deplorable. However, I believe it is important to talk about such things; after all, the purpose of this book is to encourage people with celiac disease to follow the gluten free diet and avoid the mistakes I have made in my life that caused most of these medical issues.

Finding out about the ostomy

After being educated about an ostomy, many learn that it is not as bad as they thought. It is common for the ostomy and the bag to go undetected--no one will know that you have one unless you tell them. Most importantly, having an ostomy can dramatically increase your survival, especially if the cancer is found early and treatment is provided.

Sharing the news

It can be hard to tell your friends, coworkers and loved ones that you are going to have surgery for colorectal cancer and will have to wear an ostomy bag. However, this is often approached on a need-to-know basis. For instance, there may be those who need an explanation for why you may not be able to lift heavy items anymore, or that it may be necessary to have frequent bathroom breaks for toileting needs and to manage the ostomy bag (letting air out to release trapped gas).Surgery

In some cases, surgery is performed within a few days of the diagnosis. In preparation for the surgery, the bowels will need to be cleaned out. An E.T. nurse will speak with you and your family to provide information and training about the ostomy. The ET nurse will be a valuable resource to answer questions and address any concerns about ostomy care.

The surgical course may take you from requiring pain management postoperatively, staying in bed for several days, sitting up and advancing to walking short distances, and taking a shower.

Seeing the stoma for the first time

Your stoma's healing progress will be checked by the ET nurse. It may take a few days before you are ready to look at the stoma. But, once you do, the ET nurse will be there to answer any questions.

Learning to care for the stoma

When you go home, a home health care nurse may be initially needed to provide instructions on stoma care and to provide wound care to ensure proper healing. The instructions usually include cleaning, changing the appliance, and learning what supplies to purchase and where to purchase them. Other issues, such as showering while wearing the appliance, preventing infection, and the importance of thoroughly cleaning the skin to remove all residues, are also addressed.

Daily life

Most colostomy appliances are a two-piece pouch system consisting of a flange, the portion that attaches directly to the skin, and the pouch, the portion that attaches to the flange and serves as the collecting reservoir. There are several brands to choose from on the market. Trying more than one may be necessary to find the one that works best for you.

Tips for good adherence

Preparation of the skin for good adherence of the flange is crucial to long wear time. Your skin must be clean and dried thoroughly before placing the flange. Some people have found that using a hair dryer on the lowest heat setting, or just air, dries their skin adequately. High-humidity climates and high temperatures may decrease the amount of time you can expect to wear your flange before needing to change it. A very active lifestyle and perspiration may also decrease your wear time.

Right after your surgery, you may experience problems with getting a good seal between the pouch and the flange, causing the pouch to come loose. But, in most cases after the wound around the stoma heals, it becomes easier to get a good seal.

Tips about living with the pouch

Consider always carrying an emergency kit with extra supplies such as pouches, an extra precut flange, a roll of tape, mirror, diaper wipes, and Q-tips. Wearing loose fitting tops and bottoms can help conceal your pouch in cases where you may feel self-conscious about having it hanging from your abdomen. Exercise caution when allowing your pets or young children to jump into your lap where the pouch is located. Also, be cautious when putting on your seat belt and allowing the lap belt to stretch across the area where the stoma is located.

Learning about food and digestion

Diet can be somewhat of a concern. A person with an ostomy should be especially aware of foods that cause flatulence. Of course, passing excess gas is a normal part of the digestive process, and most people typically pass gas more than 10 times a day to rid the colon of unwanted gases and pressure. The gas (a mixture of hydrogen, methane, and carbon dioxide) results from the chemical breakdown of undigested sugars in the lower intestine. Some complex carbohydrates cannot be completely broken down by normal digestive processes, and gas is the result. Altering your diet to limit these products may help. Offending foods, which vary from person to person, can include:

Asparagus

Bananas

Beans

Broccoli

Cabbage

Carbonated beverages

Carrots

Cauliflower

Dairy products (cheeses included)

Onions

Excessive amounts of fruit or fruit juice, bran, or whole-grain foods can also trigger gas. If you drink milk, try a lactose-reduced type.

Traveling tips

Pack extra ostomy supplies and, if you are flying, never pack all your supplies in the checked baggage. Limit and be aware of what you ingest before you travel.

Tips about odor

Liquid and solid products are available to help control odor. Some are placed into the pouch, while others can be taken internally. It may help to empty your pouch often as well. As for embarrassing moments, they say that anything that doesn't kill you makes you stronger. There may be times when all is quiet and your stoma decides to let out some gas.

Effect on stool

Depending on the type of surgery you have, passing of stools may occur at any time. Most often this is advantageous, seldom a detriment. Drinking plenty of water is a necessity to keep water in the stools for as long as possible while it passes through the colon. An occasional dose of a laxative may also be warranted to keep the waste softer, but check with your health care provider first before taking them. Increasing vegetables, fruits, and juices may also help. Blockage (constipation) can be a problem for someone with a colostomy. Therefore, you have to keep track of bowel movements, including their consistency and frequency.

2008 - A Mishmash Year

I continued to learn about living with my "Buddy" and became more and more active. At first, I was not sure if I would have the energy to go the one block to the store for groceries, even though I had the mobility scooter and the streets were passable. I mentioned this to Cousin Ray and he replied, "Well there is only one way to find out and that is do it!" I responded, "But what if I have a problem and can't get back home?" to which Ray replied, I will be there with you." The trip went fine and now I have more confidence and life just keeps improving!

Need a Boost?

One morning after breakfast and all the home care people had come and gone, I decided to go to the lobby to check the mail. When I opened the apartment door I encountered a stacked of Boost and Carnation Instant Breakfast! Luckily, I had a hand truck and was able to move the stack into my apartment. (I was still too weak to manhandle it) Shortly after this delivery, my dietician, Nanette, visited and we discussed my diet, Nanette suggested perhaps I should not continue with the boost as I am eating quite well and don't require the extra calories.

I didn't want to waste the Boost or cereal so I asked all my neighbors' if they would like some, and the health care aids knew people who used it, so it was soon gone.

A Nasty Fall

It was April 5th; one day before Elaine's birthday. I was over at Ken and Gail's and we were getting ready to meet our siblings for a birthday celebration in a restaurant. As I stepped down from the kitchen to the back door, I fell and gashed my left leg (shin) open right to the bone. At first I thought I had just scraped my shin but it began bleeding profusely. Gail immediately grabbed a towel and made a tourniquet while she was on the phone to 911. Within about five minutes there were three or four firemen at the door and right behind them were two paramedics. The paramedics looked at the gash, commented that Gail's actions were totally effective; helped me onto the gurney and put me in the ambulance and off we went. As we were going to the hospital, I noticed Gail was following us in her car and she stayed with me until about 8 p.m. Ken had gone to the restaurant. Everyone asked, "Where are Gail and Ron?" to which Ken replied, "Ron had to go to the hospital and I guess that Gail went with him." Elaine was very concerned. She finished her dinner and rushed to the hospital. When she arrived she asked what was happening and Gail told her about the fall and gashed shin, then asked, "Didn't Ken have dinner with you?" to which Elaine responded, "Yes, he said that Ron was in the hospital but didn't say why or what happened". Since my injury was non-life threatening, I waited until about 1 a.m. to have my wound taken care then I was on my merry way.

Another visit to the Grace hospital

One evening in June I was out and about on my scooter and began experiencing some difficulty breathing. I wasn't sure why but I wasn't very concerned about it. I returned home and went to bed. In the morning I awoke and found I was still somewhat short of breath. I assumed perhaps I was developing a cold. When Geri, a health care aid, came in she noticed my shortness of breath right away and asked, "Why am I breathing so erratically?" I told her, "I don't know" and she said, "You are going to the hospital". I called Brother Ken and asked if he would take me to the Grace Hospital. He arrived in about 20 minutes and Geri helped me out to his truck. At the hospital, Ken dropped me off at the emergency and said, "I will find a place to park and wait for you". I replied, "I don't know how long I'll be or if I will be admitted, I will call you when I know". Within a few minutes I was triaged and told I will be staying awhile for further tests. I phoned Ken and told him, "I will be in the hospital for a few hours so there would be no point in waiting". Ken replied, "I am going out to camp". (Referring to his lot in St. Laurent, Manitoba upon which he had a travel trailer).

A short time later I had a chest x-ray and was informed that I had a collapsed left lung. The nurse informed me that the E.R. Doctor will be inserting a chest tube and they would observe me to see if my lung would re-inflate. The insertion of the chest tube was extreme torture and within 30 minutes of it being inserted I was told it was in the wrong location and would require removing and reinserting. I retorted, "You have got to be kidding!" The nurse politely replied, "I am very sorry but it has to be done; Dr. P, a thoracic surgeon is on her way and she will insert the tube." Within about half an hour Dr. P and the nurse came into my cubical and removed the chest tube and began re-inserting another tube. In about 10 minutes the surgeon left the cubicle and I said in an exasperated manner, "Where is she going? ...let's get this thing done!" The nurse replied, "It is done and we will be getting another x-ray to ensure it's in the right place". I was flabbergasted as to how the first procedure was so difficult and painful while the second one was done so quickly and pain free!

When Dr. P returned to the hospital to see me, she informed me, "That since my lung had not re-inflated, it indicated there was a hole in my lung and I would require surgery to have it repaired". Surgery went well and as I convalesced, I wondered how the surgery was done as I could not see any incisions. Finally I asked a nurse and she informed me I have a large incision near my left scapula. It turned out to be a very large scar.

Since moving to Westwood, I enjoyed attending the Lyric Theater concerts in June, July and August. Ray St. Germaine was scheduled for one of the first concerts of the season while I was in the Grace Hospital. I so wanted to see the concert as I have always been a big fan of Rays. Ray was getting near the age of retirement so the opportunity of seeing his live concerts was narrowing. Of course I never got to see Ray that year but did about 2 years later with the added bonus of his son D.J. and guitarist Denis Hammerstedt.

CHAPTER SEVEN

The Elkhorn Invasion

It was a very heartwarming experience to return home to Elkhorn on August 5th, 2008. Because I was hospitalized during the 125th Elkhorn Homecoming in 2007, I could not attend. At Elaine and Dennis' request, many of my friends and our family friends agreed to return to Elkhorn in 2008, which they did.

Elaine, her daughters Michelle and Jenelle, Dennis and I headed off to Elkhorn in the early morning hours of August 5th, 2008. I was very happy to be healthy once again and looked forward to the weekend. We arrived about noon and went to the hotel, got our room keys, had some lunch and unpacked.

We then decided to take a tour of the town while we were waiting for our family friend Ernie and his wife Eileen to arrive from Saskatoon. When we returned to the hotel we noticed a car with Saskatchewan plates parked at the hotel and I wondered if it was Ernie and Eileen. I had not as yet met Eileen and had not seen Ernie since 1981. There was a lady sitting in the car so I approached to ask if they were Ernie and Eileen from Saskatoon. She said I'm Eileen and live just outside of Saskatoon but my husband's name is Norman, (Norm). I thought "What a coincidence!", then Ernie came around the corner and I recognized him immediately as he did me. We embraced and went back to his car where he introduced me to Eileen. (Afterwards, I realized Eileen was "yanking my chain", obviously, she would know Norman and Ernie is the same guy)

"Norm" is a great story teller so we had to ask how he ended up being known as Norm in Saskatchewan. It turns out that Ernie applied to the R.C.M.P. after graduating and he signed his name as Ernest Norman Greer. He was asked if that was his full legal name and he replied, "Actually my first name is Norman but everyone calls me Ernie." He was told that he would be required to go by his proper legal name. In the end, Ernie, (as I jokingly insist he be called when he visits Manitoba) attended college in Saskatoon and became a plumber; then after a number of years in the trade, he taught plumbing for 13 years. At the time of this writing, Ernie and Eileen own and live on a small ranch outside of Saskatoon. Ernie enjoys working with horses and mules; Eileen is a very accomplished artist and teaches art.

Our other friends, Betty and Al, who live in Elkhorn, came by to visit us at the hotel, as did Jackie from Virden. I asked Betty where Dennis K (a classmate) lives as I intended to look him up. She explained they were having a garage sale and gave us directions to their house. We noticed the garage sale signs as we toured the town so knew exactly where to go. We drove into Dennis' yard and he came over to the car. He did not recognize me so I said, "We heard you were having a garage sale and wanted to look around." He replied, "Sorry, we already packed everything up." We spoke for a few more minutes, then I removed my sunglasses and stepped out of the car but he still did not recognize me. I said, "You don't know who I am, do you?" He replied, "No I don't, where would I know you from?" I said, "We went to school together right from grade one through nine." Of course that didn't help so I told him my name. We shook hands, talked about how long it's been since we last saw each other, and then agreed to meet at the "Creamie" for breakfast on Sunday morning.

Ernie and Betty have summer birthdays and the plan was to celebrate their birthdays on Saturday with a steak barbecue. Betty reserved the Community Center for the barbecue. Chef Dennis was designated as chief steak burner. We went to the hall at about 4 p.m. to set up and soon other invited friends began to arrive. I had not seen my buddy Harvey (Harv) and his wife Darlene for over 25 years and was anxiously awaiting their arrival. Finally they appeared at the door and I recognized them immediately. We embraced and had a long catch up session.

Now it was time for steak and baked potatoes along with a delicious salad fresh from the garden. Everyone enjoyed their meal and by about 9:30 p.m. after much chatter we decided to clean up. Everyone was game for breakfast at the Creamie and I asked Harv if he would bring his Mom too because I had not seen her since I was seventeen; 42 years. Mom B was always very good to me and I considered her my second Mom.

It finally arrived, breakfast with all our long lost friends, and yes, Mom B came for breakfast too. Mom was 87 years of age and still as agile as ever! We all chatted while we ate our breakfast. I had a surprise visit from a classmate I hadn't seen since about 1964 or 1965. As I was eating and chatting, he came over to me and tapped me on the shoulder. When I turned I recognized Gerry L immediately. He was the headline musician for the125th Homecoming (I never knew he was musically inclined). Gerry and I weren't close personal friends but we played basketball together and generally had a mutual respect for each other. He had heard about my battle with cancer and informed me that his wife was in the hospital with cancer. Sadly, she passed away the following year.

After breakfast, we all decided to continue our visit across the street where there were some benches on the sidewalk as well as a large clock and memorial wall which was created for the 125th Homecoming the previous year. It was a nice visit with lots of chatter and photos being taken; the noon hour came before we knew it so it was time to say our good byes, pack up and head back to our real lives of 2008.

On our way, we stopped at the Manitoba Antique Auto Museum and had our lunch on the benches outside. Then we went into the museum to view the relics of the past. I feel a personal connection to the museum in two ways. When the museum was being built in 1965 or 1966, I was hired by the contractor to help pour the concrete floor. My other connection to the museum is that I knew Mr. Isaac Clarkson "Ike" personally. I recall one winter when I was helping my Dad in the welding shop; Ike asked Dad if he could use some of the equipment in the shop to make a fender for the car he was rebuilding. I was amazed when Ike went home at the end of the day with a fully formed fender. About six months later he invited us out to his farm to show us the completed car for which he made the fender. One year earlier, this car consisted only of a frame, axels and steering wheel. Ike was an exceptional car restore person.

Tribute

As a youngster Isaac "Ike" Clarkson marveled each time the 1909 Hupmobile owned by Mathew Black of Two Creeks passed by his home. Years later Mr. Clarkson, a farmer living near Elkhorn, Manitoba, purchased the remains of the very Hupmobile and set about restoring it. Replacing much of the old metal, wood and glass parts, re-upholstering it and repainting it, Clarkson was in his glory. It was 1946 and the beginning of an idea.

Ike undertook to preserve a part of Manitoba's History which might have otherwise ended up in scrap metal heaps. His genuine interest in the restoration of old cars spurred him to collecting old cars and parts, primarily from within a 200 – mile radius of his home. During his lifetime he had traveled thousands of miles gathering a variety of early makes and models which eventually became Manitoba's first antique automobile museum.

Storage did present problems. The cars were stored at the home of Marguerite Ablett whose farm Ike worked on a shared-basis. Miss Ablett supported Ike in his endeavors whenever she could. When he has accumulated some sixty cars, through purchases and donations, he offered his life's work to the Village of Elkhorn. A non-profit organization, the Manitoba Automobile Museum Foundation was realized in 1961.

For Ike his greatest dream had come true. A museum was opened in 1967 and he continued to work on the cars until his passing in 1971 at the age of 58. After Mr. Clarkson's death, Miss Ablett as the beneficiary turned over the entire estate to the museum. Today she is recognized as being a co-founder of the museum.

A cairn with a plaque has been raised in front of the museum to commemorate the two individuals for their dedication in preserving our heritage.

http:// www.mbautomuseum.com/

I encourage stepping into the past and visiting the museum if you are ever in the neighborhood of Elkhorn. It is located on Trans-Canada Highway 1 in Elkhorn, Manitoba. It has a collection of over 100 automobiles that date back to 1908. The museum has a collection of pioneer farm equipment, steam tractors, and unique household artifacts. Included in the museum's collection are: a 1904 Holsman, a 1909 Metz, a 1914 Briscoe and a 1918 Gray-Dort. The collection also includes lesser-known automobiles such as the Maxwell and the Russel-Knight.

CHAPTER EIGHT

... So Now I'm a Publisher!

With renewed friendships and no health issues, life is good! In the spring of 2009, I applied to volunteer as Publisher of Celi-Yak News, a newsletter for people with celiac disease published by the Manitoba Chapter of the Canadian Celiac Association.

I eventually "learned the ropes" of publishing the newsletter and began inputting some of my own creativity with no criticism from the executive or readers. Over time I implemented changes to the newsletter that increased the print quality while decreasing the cost of distributing the printed newsletters. As for the online copy I utilized "page flip" technology to provide a realistic read for online subscribers. Other changes include using full page bleeds and more graphics including an ever changing full page image on the cover page. The placing of advertisements was also changed to all be on the left hand pages only. Another revision was changing the cost of ads to reflect their location in the newsletter. For example, an ad on the back cover page is most prominent thus a Page Level 1 fee is applied; the inside front cover page is the second most prominent page thus a Page Level 2 fee is charged for this page and so on. The latest change implemented in 2015 was to publish the online version in an interactive format. Using this technology, the reader can have the articles read to him/her, watch videos, select and print pop-up media (coupons, etc.), watch slide shows, visit websites and much more. At the end of 2015, after a year of illnesses and unconfirmed medical diagnosis', I submitted my resignation.

Going back to 2010, the Manitoba Chapter held the National Convention in Winnipeg. I was honored with the offer of being selected as Chapter delegate and was requested to tell my story to a group of dieticians and to another group of newly diagnosed celiac patients. I am by no means a public speaker but it was important to me to get this message out, especially to the parents of celiac children, and celiac patience in general. Part of my presentation described my teen years when I would go out with my buddies, sometimes drink beer and often go for a cheeseburger at the end of the evening. I mean, after all, no self-respecting teen is going to say "no, I can't drink beer or eat hamburgers".

After presenting my story I was approached by two parents, one with a pre-teen child and another whose child was in his early teens. They both thanked me for the information and told me they had never considered the peer pressure their children would experience about drinking or eating forbidden foods. It felt good that my message did get out!

The next day I was quickly approached by an elderly lady who walked up to me and bluntly stated, "You presented a wonderful speech yesterday, we need more people like you". I was about to tell her the intention of my story was to prevent more people like me, but she turned and walked away as quickly as she arrived.

I eventually became a member of the Manitoba Chapter and remain as such at the time of this writing.

Life is good!

CHAPTER NINE

Kathleen

Now with health issues out of the way, at least for now, I thought how nice it would be if I were to meet a lady. I was concerned as to how a future mate would respond to my ostomy and all the scars from numerous surgeries, so I decided I would disclose this information in a timely manner according to the potential of our relationship.

I began poking around on the internet and tried a few mating sites before I came across "Plenty of Fish (POF). This site was free and very well set up in terms of creating a profile and being able to safely communicate with other members without giving up one's personal contact information. I communicated with several women, some were short lived and others appeared to be "possibilities". On occasion, I would meet a person online whom I felt may be compatible. If the feeling was mutual, we would agree on a public meeting place and time, thus meeting in a safe manner. Some of these meetings were a onetime thing and others involved a few dates; but the "magic" was just not there.

One evening as I was logged onto POF, a notice popped up from Kathy. This was a new one to me as Kathy did not appear on my POF. As it turned out, my search radius was 25 miles whereas Kathy, being in Pinawa, Manitoba, had a search radius which included Winnipeg.

In her profile photo, Kathy was wearing a big hat and an even bigger smile! She was beautiful!

We began emailing back and forth. I enjoyed her emails so much that when I got up in the morning, I would go to the computer to see if Kathy had emailed me. Eventually we decided to exchange phone numbers and began phoning each other. At this point, Kathy (a widow) had sold her house and had rented an apartment in Winnipeg. She traveled to Winnipeg frequently as her apartment was being remodeled to her specifications. On one occasion in late August, we agreed it was finally time to meet in person. We chose to meet at a restaurant for lunch and our first "date" was enjoyable for both of us. We agreed to see each other again. Whenever Kathy came to Winnipeg we arranged to meet. Eventually Kathy came to my apartment for lunch; on another occasion I went to Pinawa with her good friends Allen and Elda to visit Kathy.

Kathleen Elaine Huycke (nee Doyle) is an amazing lady! She is afflicted with ataxia, a mild form of Cerebral Palsy. Kathy attended the University of Winnipeg and Manitoba and after graduation taught at Emile Parochial School. In the early 1970's, this brave young lady flew off to The Pas, Manitoba, then to Moose Lake, about 74 km southeast of The Pas.

Moose Lake has an interesting history of its own. Thomas Henry Peacock Lamb (also known as THP Lamb or Ten Horse-Power Lamb) built a trading post on the western shore of Moose Lake called Lamb's Store (better known as The Post) In 1900. Moving ahead in history, THP's son, Tom Lamb, bought The Post from his father and operated it for years. Eventually, Tom's son-in-law Jock McAree and daughter Carol (Lamb) bought The Post from Tom Lamb. Jock ran the store for several years.

In 1935, Tom incorporated Lamb Airways Limited. The airline had some name changes throughout the years and Tom became one of the best known Manitobans, if not Canadians, in the world. His adventures have been documented in books, a television documentary and even a song.

From Wikipedia

Kathy, a city girl, is now in another world! In the summer, one could fly out or boat out of Moose Lake and in the winter one could fly out, go by Bombardier Snowmobile or drive on the winter road to The Pas. Jock McAree took Kathy under his wing as did Allen Havard, who at the time worked in the store. Allen and Kathy became the best of friends and to this day are very close. (Allen went on to become a teacher and for many years was the principle at the school in Ebb and Flow First Nations on the western shore of Lake Manitoba)

Kathy taught school in Moose Lake for two years. During this time she met her future husband, Brian Huycke, a social worker from The Pas. After completing her second year, Kathy moved to The Pas. It wasn't long before Kathy and Brian were married. Kathy continued teaching in The Pas. As time went on, the hard working couple met an elderly man who advised them about "preparing for their future". This plan seemed very doable to Kathy and Brian so they began investing, and as a result, were able to retire early to enjoy the fruits of their labor.

They also bought and sold several properties. Kathy really wanted to be an interior designer so enjoyed doing the interior design work on these properties. They were able to upgrade their home with each new purchase and eventually pay cash for their homes.

As if their busy lives weren't busy enough, Kathy ran for and secured a seat on The Pas town council. She remained as Counselor for nine years. Brian was elected to a four year term on the School Board.

At forty-eight, Kathy retired, mainly due to her deteriorating condition. Shortly thereafter, Brian retired and they lived comfortably on their investment incomes until they were of age to collect their pensions. During this time they took cruises and vacations to many locations around the world.

The Lower Rio Grande Valley area of Texas was a place Kathy and Brian enjoyed during the winter season. They traveled to the valley every October and returned in April. At first they rented a mobile unit, and then purchased one, then when the brick house they had their eye on came up for sale, they purchased it. They enjoyed their home for 6 years and Kathy sold it a loss.

Wedding bells are in the future!

October came and Kathy moved into her apartment. We spent a lot of time together and before Christmas, we decided to take the plunge and get married. The wedding date was set for October 23, which is also Kathy's birthday.

Kathy invited my family for Christmas dinner at her apartment in 2010 and we announced our plans to marry.

Victoria B.C. via VIA Rail

In January, Kathy and I went to Victoria on VIA Rail. It was a time of many firsts for me; my first time on a train; my first time going west of Moosomin, Saskatchewan; my first time seeing mountains and most impressive; my first time seeing no snow in January.

The trip to Victoria was a real adventure of its own. We were in Sleeper Plus class which consisted of an upper and lower bunk and a wash room and included meals meals. The train had two domed cars, one at the rear and one in the middle. The delicious meals were served in the dining room. At the time of booking this trip, we requested gluten free options. When we went to the dining room for breakfast on the first morning, I requested gluten free toast. The waiter commented, "Oh, so you're the reason we were stopped in Saskatoon in the middle of the night. We were running all over town for gluten free bread for you!" I know we were stopped somewhere for a while late in the night but I can hardly believe they were hunting for gluten free bread!

During the first day, we were invited to a beer tasting party in the rear dome car. I assumed they would not have gluten free beer so took one from the six-pack I brought with me. I explained to the bar tender that I could not drink regular beer and asked if he would open the one I brought, he quickly took it and explained, "You are not allowed to bring your own beverage but because it is a diet requirement, I will serve this to you in a glass sir." I thanked him very much and went into the seating area where we were entertained by a fellow passenger who played the violin.

The next day it was announced there would be entertainment in the middle dome car. Kathy and I made our way there to find standing room only. The lady violinist who played in the rear car the previous day had teamed up with another musician who played guitar and sang country. It was a very enjoyable show as we swayed back and forth with the train movement. Hopefully we kept in time with the music! We were then treated to a soloist country guitarist singer from Nova Scotia.

On the third day we arrived in Vancouver and were whisked away to the airport to catch our flight to Victoria. We arrived in Victoria about two o'clock in the afternoon only to find snow on the ground! We checked into our hotel and relaxed until dinner time which we ordered in.

The next day we took a cab to the grocery store and stocked up for our months stay. We found the price of groceries somewhat higher than at home in Winnipeg.

Kathy's long-time friends from Pinawa, Allan and Shirley, who were also vacationing in Victoria, came by to visit and we made plans to "tour Victoria" with them. (They drove to Victoria so had a car) We were invited on two occasions and both tours were very interesting. We learned a lot about the city and surrounding area which we were able to pass onto our friends and family at a later time.

By the way, the snow melted before the end of the first day and it never snowed again. We enjoyed average day time temperatures of $+10^C$ while back home it was in the - 30^C to -40^C range. This prairie boy was quite excited to be able to have such great weather in the middle of winter, but did not know what was in store for me for future travels!

We flew back home in early February and rejoined the Winterpeg crowd.

Now it's time to plan a wedding

Sometime in August, Elaine told me of her plans to have a bridal shower for Kathy. She asked that I get all Kathy's lady friends' contact information without asking Kathy. Well it was no small feat but I managed to make up a list and I don't think anyone was left out. Elaine called all these strangers and invited them into her home for this shower!

The day of the shower arrived and I drove Kathy to Elaine's; but Elaine wanted us to come after all Kathy's friends had arrived. We were a bit early so I drove slowly then just happened to take a wrong turn. After killing ten minutes we arrived at Elaine's just at the right time. The look on Kathy's face was priceless as she approached the living room full of her friends from Pinawa and The Pas.

We planned a small wedding inviting family and a few friends. We rented the dining room in Kathy's apartment building (Kiwanis Chateau) for the wedding celebration. Following hors d'oeuvres, a delicious rib roast dinner including potato and veggie sides was served. Kathy's wedding party consisted of her "adopted big brother" Allen (who spoke on Kathy's behalf) and his wife Esmeralda and Kathy's uncle Pat, Dr. F.P. Doyle (age 89). My wedding party was made up of Elaine (who spoke on Ron's behalf and took every opportunity to jokingly affront him), Brother Dennis and Cousin Ray. Others involved in the formality were Ron's brother Ken and Kathy's friend Bill, who witnessed the wedding. Brother Dennis was the honorary chef in charge of roasting the prime rib to perfection, and his partner Ken (also a cook) managed the wait staff and made sure everything went off without a hitch. Ron's niece, Michelle was the official photographer and her beau, Dickson, greeted the guests at the door. Both nieces, Michelle and Jenelle were ring bearers. Our guests came from all around including Winnipeg, many from Pinawa who had moved from The Pas, some new friends Kathy made in Pinawa after moving from The Pas, Portage La Prairie and Saskatoon, Saskatchewan. All the ladies wore hats in honor of Kathy as she loves hats, the bigger the better; she has a large collection of them. Even some of the male guests wore a hat … it was so much fun!

Our Honeymoon at Graceland …

We settled into a new life together with hopes of good health and a long, happy relationship. In just two short days, our hopes of good health were dashed! I suddenly had what I would say was one of the most excruciating pains I ever experienced. It was in my abdominal area, where I had much surgery in the past. Kathy took me to the Grace Hospital where I spent the night in the E.R.

After several tests it was determined the pain was caused by a ruptured gall bladder. I was told that I have a stone in my bile duct and it had to be removed before they could do surgery on my gall bladder. I was transported to the St. Boniface Hospital to have the stone removed; then back to the Grace to have my gall bladder removed. Dr. Z planned to do the surgery laparoscopically which would result in a shorter hospital stay and recovery period. When I awoke from surgery, I had a nasogastric (NG) tube in my nose. I asked several nurses why the tube was inserted and got several different answers ranging from "It is a normal procedure and ask Dr. Z". I knew it wasn't normal procedure and when Dr. Z visited the next morning he explained that because my colon was adhering to the front of my abdomen it did not show up on the ultrasound and when he put the camera in to begin the surgery he punctured my colon (hence the nasogastric tube) thus he had to do the surgery using a scalpel. This resulted in a twelve day hospital stay instead of a 3 or 4 day stay. So, when folks ask, we spent our twelve day honeymoon at Graceland!

The problems just kept coming!

When we returned from our "honeymoon", all went well for a short time, and then I started experiencing blockages (bowel obstructions). I would have a very uncomfortable swelling in my abdominal area, near the stoma, and on most occasions I would begin to vomit large amounts over a period of up to 8 to 12 hours. On these occasions it would take me a week or longer to regain my strength. On occasion, when I had an obstruction, I would go to the E.R. as advised by the E.T. Nurses but in every case I was observed for 8 to 10 hours and sent home without treatment. On one such visit, a nurse implied that I needed to stay on my gluten free diet then I wouldn't be unnecessarily visiting the E.R. I simply replied, "There is not one gluten containing food in our home except for one loaf of wheat based bread which my wife eats."

Around this period of time, our family doctor closed his practice and referred us to a new clinic that was just opening. We visited the clinic and were directed to one of the doctors. This doctor was a very recent graduate but seemed undaunted by my medical history and agreed to become our family doctor. Sometime after, I was feeling quite "sickly" with an upset stomach, fever and dehydration. We called our new doctor and were able to visit her that day. As I was sitting in her office, I was shaking and very thirsty. I asked her if I could get a glass of water to which she replied, "You can buy a bottle of water at the drug store next door." She provided me with a subscription for an ant-acid (Pepto-Bismol) and Dimenhydrinate (Gravol™). We purchased the medications and as Kathy was driving back home, I took the medication as prescribed, but by the time we arrived home I vomited it all up.

My condition continued to worsen so we decided I should go to the E.R at the Grace Hospital. When we arrived, I went into the E.R. while Kathy parked the car. As soon as I stepped in the door, the Triage Nurse rushed over and seated me in a wheel chair and pushed me into the back of the E.R. I told her I had not been triaged to which she replied "There is no time for that right now, we will do that after we get you stabilized." I knew I wasn't feeling well but did not realize I was so seriously ill.

I was immediately surrounded by nurses who took my vitals and started an IV. I was informed that I have no blood pressure and am severely dehydrated. After about an hour, I was moved to another part of the E.R. where a doctor took over my care. He explained that he needed to get my blood pressure back up as he attached two IV infusion pumps and began pumping fluids into me at a very rapid rate.

He worked on me all night and by 7 a.m. he declared my blood pressure was within a safe range. Now it was time to diagnose what was causing these problems. I had an x-ray and later an ultrasound. Sometime later, as I lay dozing on the gurney, my old friend, Dr. DI came by and woke me. He said, "Ron, even though your gall bladder was removed last year, as strange as it may sound, you have another gall stone which we think is causing your symptoms. We are going to send you to St. Boniface to have the stone removed, and then we'll get you back here for observation." After three days of observation, my symptoms disappeared and my vitals returned to normal, so I was discharged.

As I continued to experience obstructions, Kathy would frequently look for causes on the internet. On one research session, Kathy found a site that recommended peeling all fruits and vegetables. We began peeling everything that was peel able, and avoid other foods that were not so easily peeled, such as grapes. It worked! I stopped having frequent blockages. I have had an occasional "soft" blockage; that is my stoma would become overwhelmed (from me eating too much) so I would stop eating for a day and drink lots of fluids including meal replacement drinks. My stoma would slowly empty in a normal manner and I could recover within a day.

CHAPTER TEN

Elkhorn Revisited

We're off back home to Elkhorn again. Our entourage included Kathy, Dennis, our brother Ken and me. Unfortunately, sister Elaine did not go due to booking mix-ups with an Alaskan Cruise. Dennis, Kathy and I went in our van and Ken drove his truck.

This time we planned to stay in Virden and drive back and forth to Elkhorn everyday but the issue of drinking came up (we do enjoy a few bottles of (gluten free) beer and glasses of wine now and then) and there is no better time or place than with good friends. For that reason, we decided to rent a motor home and stay at the campground. We rented a 24 foot motorhome from a RV company in Brandon.

We arrived in Brandon and after one wrong turn, we called the RV Company for directions and arrived at their site shortly after. We did our business and got on the road again. Now our convoy consisted of Kathy in the van, me in the RV and Ken taking up the rear. About 1 hour later we arrived in Elkhorn. Dennis and Ken were going to stay at the hotel so Kathy stopped there and I went on to the campground with the RV.

I drove into the campground past rows of high priced motorhomes from Alberta. As I got to our reserved site, Betty and Al were busy erecting a dining tent. We said our hellos and embraced, and then I backed the RV into our spot and hooked up the electrical and water.

Later we had lunch and Betty joined us in the RV. I asked Betty about all the RV's from Alberta, she replied, "They are all oil pipeline workers. They are setting up multiple oil pumps just south of Elkhorn". I recall in the early 60's, oil companies were drilling exploratory wells all over the Elkhorn area for several years. I often wondered why they would spend so much money and time if they were not finding oil. I realize now they were oil reserves and waiting for the oil prices to become more profitable before they began extracting the black gold.

As the day went on, I asked Betty if she knew Larry and Wendy Price. She said, "Not personally, but there is a Price in the first lot near the entrance. I wondered over and sure enough, it's my old buddy Larry and his wife Wendy. We visited for a while then I returned to our site as Ernie had pulled in and I went to greet them and help with setting up his rig next to our RV.

Larry, Wendy and I met later that evening at the registration and meet and greet. We mingled and met a number of people I had not seen since school days.

On Saturday we invited Dennis for breakfast as Ken was going to Virden. As it turns out, Ken went to the Creamee Restaurant for breakfast so Dennis went with him; then Ken drove Dennis to the campground before going to Virden.

Later on in the afternoon, folks drifted in and out of our camp to visit. "Ole Arnie" stopped by once or twice and Larry and Wendy dropped by. I introduced them to Kathy and we spent some time catching up and getting to know each other. I was quite amazing how Larry, Wendy and I reconnected as if there were no 35 year time-lapse; and how well they connected with Kathy in such a short time.

Soon it was time to go for dinner at the curling rink. The self-serve meal was a bit bland but the people were grand! At one point Dennis called Kathy and I over to meet Pat. Pat was our neighbor across the street, and her Mom was our early grade school teacher. Pat pointed in the direction of her Mom and I could not believe my eyes; I recognized Mrs. R immediately!

Kathy and I walked toward Mrs. R and as we approached, I held my hand over my I.D. tag. Mrs. R, who was in her early nineties, didn't miss a beat, she said, "I remember you Ronnie Webster!"

We finished our dinner and visiting and headed back to our camper. Everyone was everywhere around Elkhorn. There was a dance scheduled for later in the evening which we didn't plan to attend as we were saving our energy for the Sunday evening street dance featuring my former class mate, Gerry.

Sunday morning arrived and I was anxious for what seemed to be a budding tradition, cow boy breakfast cooked over the fire. Everyone brought a breakfast ingredient and we all pitched in to make a delicious breakfast over the fire. Dennis and Ernie cooked the scrambled eggs, delicious thick maple bacon and sausages imported from Saskatoon, Saskatchewan; I cut up the potatoes and Al grilled them up on the barbeque. It was a very enjoyable feast indeed!

Throughout the day, folks drifted in and out the camp and visited. Some went visiting old friends around town or to the horse show that was taking place in the nearby fair grounds.

Soon it was dinner time and Kathy and I had dinner, then prepared for the much anticipated street dance. Kathy wore a cowboy hat, jacket and jeans with her sharp towed cowgirl boots. She was striking! I wanted "to go back to the day" so I wore a white t-shirt, blue jeans and leather jacket. I tried to buy Brylcreem™ to finish off the look but couldn't find any, so I settled for a very stiff gel which did the trick.

We drove downtown and sat near the curb close to the music. Gerry had a big motorhome as a background to their stage and soon they started the show. I was somewhat disappointed that it was a different than that of 2007. Back in '07, Gerry did a lot of Rock-n-Roll and Elvis while his lady singer "did an excellent Patsy Cline" as Dennis described it.

As darkness fell, there was an exciting display of pyrotechnics put on by Archangel Fireworks from Winnipeg.

On Monday morning, the mood was somber as it was the day to say our good byes and head back to our everyday lives. With each gathering, it gets harder to say good bye as we never know when or if we will meet again.

Life is even better than good!

CHAPTER ELEVEN

Rendezvous at the Grace

As it was in 2007, Dennis and I were about to have surgery again at the same time. This time, Dennis' surgery will be in the Grace Hospital and mine will be at the Health Sciences Center (HSC)

Dennis' surgery involved a urostomy while I was to have the right upper lobe of my lung removed, laparoscopically. Of all the surgeries I have had to date, this was my first laparoscopic surgery. I was experiencing good health at this time and there were no concerns about my surgery. I had the surgery on Thursday afternoon and by Saturday morning I was discharged from the HSC.

On the following Monday I visited Dennis at the Grace. He looked at me and said, "I thought you were going to have surgery?" to which I replied, "I did." Dennis could not believe I was mobile and feeling so well so soon.

Dennis soon recovered and was discharged. As it was with me having an ostomy, now Dennis has to learn how to live with his urostomy. I was glad that I had the experience and was able to help Dennis with his.

Once Dennis was home, his partner, Ken, Kathy and I teamed up to give Dennis the care he required. The first thing I did was go to the Health Sciences Center (HSC) Materials Handling to get Dennis' urostomy supplies. Things seemed to go well after Dennis' return home. For the rest of the year Dennis attended countless doctor appointments and medical tests.

A Triple Tragedy

As time went on Dennis' health deteriorated. Shortly before Christmas he was admitted into the Grace hospital where he remained until after Christmas. This year it was Dennis and Ken's turn to host Christmas. In spite of the family's offers to host Christmas, Ken insisted he would do it. On Christmas morning, before going to Dennis and Ken's apartment, Kathy and I went to see Dennis at the Grace. He was in his usual jovial mood and was eating the "Graceland" version of Christmas dinner. He laughed as he cut into a ball of dressing saying "this is supposed to be dressing but it looks more like road apples!" Back at Dennis and Ken's apartment, the festive mood was dampened but everyone acknowledged Dennis' spirits were up when they heard about the road apple comment. Dennis was discharged shortly after Christmas only to return his regiment of doctor's appointments and medical tests.

On February 4th, 2013, we took Dennis back to the Grace Hospital Emergency. I remember this date very clearly. As we were waiting for Dennis to be taken into the Emergency Room (ER), my cell phone rang and it was our cousin Ray. When I answered I knew something was wrong, Ray was not his usual joking self. Ray asked where I was, and then dropped the bomb. He said, "Sharon passed away yesterday." Sharon was Ray's wife of over forty years.

Dennis was admitted to the hospital. His health began to deteriorate rapidly and was transferred to the Intensive Care Unit (ICU). We were all prepared for the worst but Dennis, being the fighter he was, recovered well enough to return to his former ward. He was frequently transported to St. Boniface hospital for treatments and on March 22, we received a phone call from the Grace Hospital telling us he is at the St Boniface Hospital and would be for most of the day. A few minutes later the same nurse called back to tell us St. Boniface had just called and advised the family to come to the hospital. Dennis passed peacefully around 3 p.m. that day.

About two weeks after Dennis' April 5th memorial, we received word that our only remaining aunt, Aunt Eunice passed away in Gladstone, Manitoba.

A Quick Get-A-Way

On December fourth, Kathy and I embarked on a two week vacation to the Excellence Playa Mujeres (EPM) near Cancun Mexico. We had to fly to Toronto, then to Cancun. The Cancun airport was flooded with people lined up to go through immigration and when we finally got to the Immigration clerk's desk, we were told the form was incomplete so must complete it and get back in line again. Finally we got through immigration, now we have to find our luggage and go through security and customs. I needed to go to the washroom so while there, Kathy was able to locate our luggage, half way across the airport! But now I don't know where she is; I asked an attendant for help but he did not speak English very well. Another attendant noticed I was getting distressed and asked if I needed help.

He spoke and understood English and soon I found myself in a wheel chair whisking through the crowd. I explained I didn't need a wheel chair to which he replied, "We can get you through the airport quicker." So I just sat back and relaxed. He took me right to where Kathy was guarding our luggage. Our new friend and his friend teamed up and got us through security, then customs customs and out to our waiting shuttle in double quick time!

Finally we arrived at the EPM and were greeted by Carlos with a cool, wet face cloth and a warm "welcome home." We were each served a sparkling glass of Champagne and were escorted off to our room. It was about nine in the evening and we were both "wiped" from our long day of travel. We got comfortable and browsed the room menu for some dinner. We found a nice steak dinner which we both ordered along with some white wine and red wine. The dinner was delicious after which we each had a glass of wine and retired our weary bones into bed for a good night's sleep.

In the morning, we still had jetlag so ordered breakfast and just relaxed and enjoyed the beautiful view from the balcony for the rest of the morning.

By lunch time we were rested and anxious to explore this beautiful resort. We wondered out and found a restaurant for lunch; then we wondered around the resort before returning to our room.

The next morning we were up and at it by eight A.M. and went to the restaurant for breakfast. Then we walked down to the beach and I saw the Caribbean Sea for the first time! We went on the beach and sifted sand through our toes as I thought, "Wow, it is -30^C back home and we're here on the beach enjoying $+25^C$ temperatures with a nice cool breeze from the ocean. We wondered up from the beach to the SOL Bar where Kathy had a Pina Colada and at the request of my sister I slurped on a Margarita for her.

Later we wondered around the rest of the resort, then went back to our room to relax. We decided to order some wine which was delivered by Hector. As he left our room he said, "If you need anything at all, just call me, Hector, I'm your protector!"

That evening we went to The Grill Restaurant for dinner. This was an intimate dining experience with low lighting levels in an open air dining room located over a river. We had a delicious steak dinner as we relaxed in this tranquil setting.

The next morning we went for breakfast and wondered around the resort, taking in the sights and stopping for occasional refreshments. We went for lunch and then dinner at the Barcelona. We returned to our room and shortly after Kathy retired for the night. I went onto the balcony with the tablet and connected on Skype with Elaine. We chatted for a while then I realized I needed to change "Buddy". I finished up and decided to go to bed. Within about half an hour, I began coughing and it got worse and could not stop. I sat up which helped but when I lay down again the cough returned. By about eleven P.M. Kathy called the hotel doctor who came and advised that I go to the hospital in Cancun.

Upon arriving at the hospital, the clerk took all the pertinent information then I was wheeled into an examination room. Shortly thereafter a doctor came in and asked about my medical history. He then ordered some blood work and an x-ray. I returned from the x-ray and waited in the room. I asked the nurse where Kathy was and she told me in the doctor's office. Later, Kathy came into my room with a very unhappy look on her face. She told me the doctor says I am very sick and need to be hospitalized. He explained I have acute bronchitis. We were quite certain that acute bronchitis wasn't as serious as the doctor claimed, thus opted to leave the hospital and go back to EPM to prepare to fly home on the next available flight. We were given prescriptions for anti-biotics and cough syrup which we got at a drugstore on our way back to EPM. I took the medication and returned to bed.

After numerous phone calls, Kathy had our return flight booked and the flight change fee was waived by the nice folks at West Jet. Saturday morning we headed off to the airport to fly home.

When I woke up Sunday morning I was feeling much better. My coughing had long subsided and I had more energy. I realized that we could have stayed in our room at the EPM for 2 or 3 days rather than flying home early - but it is smart to err on the side of caution.

I visited my doctor on the third day after returning home and her examination and x-ray came up with nothing; she said, "Assuming it was bronchitis, the anti-biotics that were prescribed were clearly the right ones." It was a sweet but short trip!

Christmas 2013 was celebrated at Elaine and Leo's. On this occasion Elaine made an honorary place setting in memory of Dennis at the dinner table. It was a very much appreciated gesture, although somewhat formidable.

CHAPTER TWELVE

Life Goes On

It's now January 2014. We are all filled with hopes of a happier and healthier new year.

Kathy and I planned a month get-a-way from the brutal Manitoba winter in Victoria, B.C. This would be our second trip to Victoria but this one promised to be a much more enjoyable holiday. Even though our room at the hotel we previously stayed in was reserved, we were not advised they would be closed for renovations for the period of our stay until shortly before our departure. We both began scouring the internet for another suitable hotel. It was looking grim, either the location wasn't suitable or the amenities were not as required. Then, after a few hours of googling, I decided to look at the details of the Victoria Regent Waterfront Hotel. This was the first hotel I looked at but dismissed it with the assumption that it would be priced in the $500 plus per night range. To our surprise, it was well over $1000 less than the other hotel; it was much bigger, right on the waterfront and offered a free daily continental breakfast, free underground parking and the location couldn't be better!

On the day our great adventure was to begin, we got up early and Elaine whisked us to the airport. It was a cold, blustery day and we hoped we could get off the ground before the weather got much worse. After jumping through all the hoops we went to the gate for our flight to Calgary where we would catch a connection to Victoria. When we got to the gate our flight was delayed by 20 minutes. We watched intently but lady luck was with us, the flight was not further delayed and we rose above the weather and onward to warmer places. Our next concern was that we would be rushed to catch the connecting flight to Victoria but lady luck stayed with us all through the trip! Upon disembarking in Calgary, we learned the connecting flight was coming out of Saskatoon and was also delayed 20 minutes so, in essence, we were right on time! To add to our good fortune, we found a restaurant within a few feet of our departure gate so we went for lunch and enjoyed a celebratory glass of wine to toast to a perfect start to our latest adventure. Our plane arrived and departed as expected and soon we found ourselves in Victoria on a beautiful, warm (10°C) sunny afternoon.

Shortly we arrived at the much anticipated Victoria Regent Water Front Hotel and Sean greeted us at the curb. I immediately noticed he had an Australian accent, and I have a theory that Australians, for the most part, have a great sense of humor. As Sean loaded our luggage onto the cart, I pretended to look around as though I was lost. I asked Sean, "Where are we?" He looked at me with an odd facial expression and replied, "You're in Victoria, B.C. and this is the Victoria Regent Hotel, you have reservations with us." I replied, "We are booked at the Empress Hotel, would you please take our luggage over there?" In response to his facial expression, I quickly added, "I'm just kidding!" Sean replied, "I was going to call you a cab." I answered, "Well, I don't think there is any need for name calling here!" Sean was indeed amused and soon we were taken to our beautiful water front suite which faced west. As the warm sunshine streamed in through the balcony doors, we could not resist sitting on the balcony overlooking the beautiful Victoria Harbor with a glass of wine to celebrate the beginnings of a picture-perfect holiday!

Our suite included a kitchenette, 2 large bedrooms, each with its own ensuite. The two bedrooms and living room all had full width glass with access to the balcony from each room. A complimentary breakfast buffet is provided at the hotel's Water's Edge Café located on the main floor featuring expansive windows to give a picturesque view of Victoria's Inner Harbor.

One bedroom was locked and when we inquired about it, we were told our rate included only one bedroom but if we wanted the use of both bedrooms, it would be an additional $40 per night. Kathy, knowing that Elaine and Leo were coming, went to the front desk and negotiated the rate to $30 per night. She cited, "You cannot rent the bedroom anyway while we are occupying the suite."

Since we planned to go shopping for groceries the next day, we decided to order our dinner from a restaurant. Right across from the hotel is The Joint Pizza which offers gluten free options. I couldn't wait! I got on the phone and ordered two pizzas. This was the first pizza I had for several years and I enjoyed it immensely!

The next day, we ordered a taxi and went grocery shopping. We were familiar with Thrifty Foods on Simcoe Street so went there.

There were many gluten free options as well a very good selection of fresh seafood - such a treat!

Kathy and I had settled in and we were enjoying the beautiful weather. Every morning we would go to the Water's Edge Café for breakfast. They offered no gluten free options so I would take my own bread or cereal and round out my breakfast with the cafés yogurt, fruit coffee, etc.

Wasn't that a (birthday) party!

On January ninth (my 65th birthday) Kathy asked, "What would you like for breakfast." Assuming we were going to the Café I jokingly replied, "Steak, eggs and toast with jam." I added, "I'm going to do my morning ritual (in the bathroom) and will be back in a few minutes". Well to my surprise and delight, Kathy cooked a steak and eggs, and made toast for my birthday breakfast! What a Sweetie! But this wasn't the only surprise she had for me on this day!

About 10:30 that morning, someone knocked on our door. I commented to Kathy, "The room attendant has already been here so I wonder who it would be?" Kathy replied, "I think the only way you will know who it is and what they want is to open the door!" I decided Kathy's solution was a good one and I opened the door only to see my sister Elaine and her hubby Leo. Wow, what a surprise! I could hardly believe it as Elaine and I embraced. My sixty-fifth birthday, one I never expected to see, was shaping up to be the best birthday ever! Later Elaine and Leo said, "We are treating you to a birthday dinner where ever you want to go." I replied there is a restaurant two blocks over on Wharf Street (just down the street from the hotel) called *Nautical Nellies*. They serve steaks and seafood and appear to have very good reviews. Well, the reviews were correct; the steak was cooked to perfection as was the lobster tail. We also enjoyed some sides such as alligator bites and oysters! After dinner, the waitress brought out a slice of gluten free cake with a lit candle as the wait staff sang happy birthday! Now, wasn't that a party!

The Tourists

Elaine and Leo planned to stay a week so we organized some tours and sites to see. We ventured out from the Hotel on foot to tour the neighborhood, and then on Sunday we hired a cab to give us a tour of Victoria's sites. One thing I wanted to show Elaine and Leo is the statue of Terry Fox at Mile 0.

Another site was Beacon Hill Park where flocks of ducks and peacocks abound amongst the beautiful big trees throughout the park. We followed along the shoreline and visited the Governor General's residents as well as the Craigdarroch Castle. Then we visited the Empress Hotel and walked around on the main floor. From there we walked along the Inner Harbor from the Empress to the Victoria Regent.

It turns out that Victoria is a celiac foodie's delight. Restaurants are all over the downtown area and many offer gluten free options. I researched many restaurants offering gluten free food in Victoria with the purpose of going to specific ones that offer "hard to get" food items, such as cheeseburgers.

On one of our walking adventures we stopped at the Bard and Banker Scottish Pub. They had gluten free options on the menu including beer. Their burger menu offered a gluten free option so I ordered a gluten free cheeseburger. The waitress told me the buns are gluten free, but burger patties are not gluten free. Well, what a disappointment; I wonder who thought up this option! I ordered bangers and mash which was quite tasty and soothed my disappointment somewhat!

Down the street about a block or two was the Irish Times Pub, apparently owned and managed by the same company as Bard and Banker. On our way by, we stepped in and inquired if they have gluten free burgers and they assured us they do, "We have gluten free beer too." the manager added.

Our next tour was in Chinatown..

The Chinatown in Victoria, British Columbia is the oldest Chinatown in Canada and the second oldest in North America after San Francisco's. Victoria's Chinatown had its beginnings in the mid-nineteenth century in the mass influx of miners from California to what is now British Columbia in 1858. It remains an active place and continues to be popular with residents and visitors, many of whom are Chinese-Canadians. Victoria's Chinatown is now surrounded by cultural, entertainment venues as well as being a venue itself.

Fan Tan Alley is an alley in Victoria, British Columbia's Chinatown. It runs south from Fisgard Avenue to Pandora Avenue in the block between Government Street and Store Street. It was originally a gambling district with restaurants, shops, and opium dens. Today it is a tourist destination with many small shops including a barber shop, art gallery, Chinese cafe, apartments and offices. It is the narrowest street in Canada. At its narrowest point it is only 0.9 meters (35 in) wide. It was designated as a heritage property by the local government in 2001.

http://www.tourismvictoria.com/

Unfortunately, after visiting two or three restaurants I could not find one that could assure me of their food being gluten free. One manager remarked that he thought there was only a little bit of gluten in some of the dishes so I exited stage right pronto!

Aside from the restaurant disappointment, Chinatown in Victoria is a worthwhile site to see. There are countless little shops in Tin Pan Alley and beyond. Most products are made in China and uniquely reflect the Chinese culture. One of the shopkeepers told us about their New Year's celebration and encouraged us to come back if we were still in Victoria mid-February. Unfortunately we were only there until the end of January.

We disappointedly trundled off from our visit to Chinatown; I think Leo in particular was disappointed as he loves Chinese food, as do I. We made our way back to Wharf Street with the idea of going to The Joint Pizza restaurant. Kathy and I were quite tired from our walking tour so we returned to the hotel while Elaine and Leo headed off to more adventures.

The week went by very quickly. On the eve of Elaine and Leo's departure for home, we had a steak and lobster tail dinner. Kathy cooked the dinner but asked Leo, a big barbecue fan, to cook his and Elaine's steak to their liking.

After one last breakfast at the Water's Edge Café, Elaine and Leo readied their luggage and we went to the lobby to wait for the airport shuttle. Soon they were off and we returned to our quiet life, for a few days.

Visitors From Far in the Past

Since we had the extra bedroom with ensuite we decided to invite Wendy and Larry to visit for a few days. They live near Calgary so it was just a short jaunt on the plane to come to Victoria.

On the day of their arrival I waited outside the hotel to watch for them so as to get them into the underground parking. After a few minutes I saw Wendy walking down the sidewalk across the road so I went over to her. They had been past the hotel but missed the sign which is mounted high up on the building and not easily seen from a vehicle passing by the hotel.

We walked about a half block to where Larry was parked. We drove into the parkade and brought their luggage up to the room. Once they were settled in, we ordered some bubbly from a nearby liquor store and sat and reminisced (for Kathy it was a get-to-know them session). It was absolutely amazing how, with the exception of seeing Wendy and Larry briefly in Elkhorn two years earlier, we were able to pick up where we had left off some thirty plus years earlier. Our friendship was as strong as ever, and within a few short days, Kathy felt a kinship with Wendy and Larry too.

That evening, Wendy and Larry invited us to dinner "wherever you want to eat". We mentioned that on my birthday we had visited Nautical Nellies just down the street, "and if you like steak and sea food, I recommend that restaurant". So we're off to Nautical Nellies again!

Throughout the next few days we toured Victoria and surrounding area in Wendy and Larry's rental car. We went shopping for groceries on one excursion which turned into a merry-go-round! We got onto the wrong street and in order to get back to the right one we went in here, out there and literally went round and round until we found the right street. Poor Larry got razzed for that one!

As with all good things, it was time for Wendy and Larry to return home. On the evening before their departure, Kathy and I cooked up a steak and lobster tail dinner and toasted to good friends. After breakfast the next morning, Larry and I took down the luggage and loaded it into the car. When it was time to go, we all went down to the parkade and said our good byes.

We keep in touch through Facebook and the occasional phone call. In 2014 we got a surprise call from Larry. They were in Winnipeg Beach visiting his sister and were about to leave. Larry asked if we could meet at the Headingly Husky because they had their camper and didn't want to drive through the city with it. We arrived at the Husky station and circled the parking lot looking for Larry's white truck and trailer but they weren't there! We drove past a shiny new motorhome that had a Cadillac SUV in tow and as we passed by the Caddy, there was Larry inside fiddling with something. Larry laughed as we told him we were looking for his white truck and trailer. He said, "We decided to trade in the trailer and try a motorhome for travelling; maybe take it into the southern states next winter. The motor home, which they call George, is beautiful and homey. Again we said our goodbyes and looked forward to our next visit.

The next visit came to be in November, 2015. Larry is a real Stampeders football fan and CFL nut. He attends every Grey Cup all across Canada. In 2015 the Grey Cup was held in Winnipeg and Larry, with his Grey Cup buddy, came to Winnipeg to participate in all the festivities. As it turned out, their hotel was only three blocks from our apartment. We spoke on the phone during the weekend and on Monday, Larry walked over to our apartment and we visited for about four hours. On Tuesday morning I drove them to the airport and once more said our goodbyes. (One never knows if and when "we meet again")

Our next encounter was with Kathy's "baby" brother, Tim. Tim lives and works in Victoria. Kathy phoned him and made plans to come to our suite at the Victoria Regent for lunch. It was my first meeting with Tim which turned out to be very enjoyable. Tim is quite knowledgeable about Victoria and told us about of much of its history.

The day before we were leaving, we invited Tim to have lunch with us at the Irish Times Pub. I was determined to have gluten free cheese burger before we went home. Tim came over and parked in the parkade, and then we walked to the Irish Times Pub.

I was elated to find a large menu of "pub food" that was or could easily be served sans gluten. Since I had my mouth set for a cheese burger, I ordered the Irish Bacon and Brie Burger; a grilled beef patty topped with Irish bacon and melted brie with red relish and mayo on a gluten free bun. Not only did I have a delicious hamburger, I had an Omission beer which was the best gluten free beer I had ever tasted. Sadly, it turns out that because it is made from barley with the gluten removed, the Canadian Celiac Association and Canada Food and Drug Agency do not recognize the tests offered by the U. S. brewer thus do not recommend it for consumption by celiac patients in Canada.

The one beer I had did not result in any obvious damage to my digestive system but I will avoid these kinds of beers until it is proven with absolute certainty it is safe for consumption by celiac patients.

Upon leaving the Irish Times Pub, Tim took us to a bakery just down the street. He obviously was a well-known customer and requested the staff to point out to me all the gluten free products they produce. It was quite an array but all the wheat based and gluten free products were displayed together in the display case. I wondered about their bake shop; perhaps they bake both products in the same area thus causing cross contamination. Needless to say, I didn't buy any goodies from this bakery.

We returned back to our suite, said our good byes to Tim and began preparing to return home. It was a memorable month; the gorgeous harbor view from our suite, a sixty-fifth birthday celebration with my sister and brother-in-law, a rendezvous with good friends from way in the past and a visit with Kathy's brother who was a new brother-in-law to me. This was a holiday of everlasting memories!

Life is good!

CHAPTER THIRTEEN

Fun, Sun and Surgery

Summer was "normal" and enjoyable. We attended Wednesday concerts at the Air Canada Park on Carlton Street and Portage Avenue On two occasions we met with brother-in-law Ken and once Elaine attended with us; each time coming back to our suite for lunch. We entertained in our new balcony enclosure and did what older retired folks do.

On a routine follow-up with my thoracic surgeon in October, I was told that I have another "lesion" in my right lung. I was then scheduled for a PET scan and Pulmonary function test.

A PET scan is a nuclear medicine imaging test that uses a form of radioactive sugar to create images of body function and metabolism. PET imaging can be used to evaluate normal and abnormal biological function of cells and organs.

PET uses a radiopharmaceutical made up of a radioactive isotope attached to a natural body compound, usually glucose. The radiopharmaceutical concentrates in certain areas of the body and is detected by the PET scanner.

The PET scanner is made up of a circular arrangement of detectors. These detectors pick up the pattern of radioactivity from the radiopharmaceutical in the body. A computer analyzes the patterns and creates 3-dimensional colour images of the area being scanned. Different colours or degrees of brightness on a PET image represent different levels of tissue or organ function.

PET scan machines are expensive to buy and operate, so they are not readily available. This test is only available at a very limited number of centers in Canada.

Canadian Cancer Society

My PET scan and Pulmonary function test were scheduled for 24th of December. We had a 2 month vacation booked for Cozumel in January and February 2015. Our quandary was that if the PET scan proved positive, I would be having more surgery sometime early in the New Year. We described the situation to Kathy's uncle (a medical doctor) and asked his advice. He advised that, "Since the discovery of the lesion was made in October and the PET scan is not until late December, it appears to not be an emergency situation." We decided to make an appointment to see the surgeon early in February; go on our vacation for one month, then come home at the end of January.

Cozumel - Here We Come!

On January third, we flew to and stayed overnight in Toronto. The next morning we flew to Cozumel, arriving about two p.m. We went through Immigration then went to the luggage carousel to retrieve our luggage. When the luggage stopped coming we still didn't have ours. Kathy found a WestJet representative who took our information and assured us she would locate our luggage and get it back to us.

On this trip our flights and hotel bookings did not jive well so we stayed in the Hotel Plaza in Cozumel and moved to the Cozumel Palace the next day.

We boarded our shuttle with one suitcase and headed off to the Hotel Plaza. We went in, got our room key and went up to the room. It was a nice room including two bedrooms, bathroom and a kitchenette. The view from the bedroom window was spectacular. Looking over the roof tops, we could see the Caribbean Sea. There was a pirate ship which I had spotted from the plane that was anchored off shore.

Our first concern was to try to get a WestJet representative in Toronto which we did via Skype on out tablet, and then we lost the signal and could not reconnect. We tried Skyping Elaine which we were able to do and gave her the phone number for WestJet in Canada, and the details. She phoned on our behalf but was informed they could not give her any information without our consent. We decided to carry on with the hope that our luggage would soon arrive.

Since we had a short four hour, thirty minute flight, we were still energized and went off to see some of this beautiful island. We had chosen to go to Guido's for dinner that evening, but first wanted to get a bottle of wine to take back to our room. We needed to go to the Mega Store for the wine so we got a taxi to take us, then over to Guido's, which was only two blocks from the Hotel Plaza.

When we stepped into Guido's, we were met by a waiter who took our name and informed us our wait would be about twenty minutes. We sat in the bar area and each had a margarita. We were then guided to the outdoor patio and seated. It was dark out now and the patio offered a warm, relaxing ambiance. We were provided menus and offered "a drink before dinner folks …?" We requested a glass of wine and asked if they offer gluten free options. "Indeed we do señor," replied the waiter as he pointed out the past options. We both opted for Carbonara with lobster tail. Our dinner was delicious and now it's time to go back to our room and settle in for the night.

Upon exiting Guido's, we found ourselves disorientated and decided to get a taxi so we don't get too lost. We flagged down a taxi and asked to be taken to the Hotel Plaza. I told the driver, "We are going to the Hotel Plaza". He replied, "The Cozumel Palace?" I repeated, "The Hotel Plaza, it's very close to here." He didn't seem to know where it was but it is quite popular so I assumed he just wanted to make a few extra pesos. As we drove along the water front, I spotted the Pirate ship and informed the driver that we could see the ship from our hotel room so the hotel has to be one or two blocks inland. He continued driving toward the Cozumel Palace on Av Rafael E. Melgar. Finally I told him to turn around or stop and let us out. He turned around and went two blocks inland and drove back toward Guido's. He continued to seemingly not know where the Hotel Plaza was so I asked him to stop at a drug store on Av Lic Benito Juárez.

This was very convenient because I had gotten some type of bacteria in my eye so we went into the drugstore. The pharmacist did not speak much English and I don't speak Spanish so I showed her my eye. She knew immediately what medication I required and provided me with a tube of cream for $100 pesos.

We exited the drugstore and instinctively began walking toward the water. After one block we came to 5a Avenida Sur and Kathy spotted Wet Wendy's Bar. She said, "The hotel is just around the corner from Wet Wendy's, I know this from all the Googling I have been doing about Cozumel." Sure enough, we went around the corner and half a block away, there it was, the Hotel Plaza!

The next morning we went down stairs for a complimentary breakfast. We sat on the patio in front of the hotel and enjoyed our breakfast. A bakery is located next door to the hotel and wafts of fresh baked buns drifted by as we watched the locals go in and out of the bakery. It's a seemingly quiet, laid back community, until the nightlife rouses the party animals.

Today was the day to move to the Cozumel Palace, but not until at least noon or later. We went up to the roof of the hotel where there is a bar and a swimming pool. The bar appears to be for special events and the pool appeared to be open to the public, although not promoted as such. There were a few folks coming and going, mostly locals with their children.

We're off to the Palace

The entrance to the Cozumel Palace is marked with a row of potted, baby palm trees, and friendly doormen greet guests on arrival and usher them through a set of sliding glass doors. Stepping in from the Cozumel heat, the expansive lobby provides a cool and welcoming space where polished marble floors combine with wicker furnishings and a wood-paneled reception desk to create a colonial-chic aesthetic. Cool towels and drinks on arrival are a nice touch, the time-share marketing less so. The vibe however is generally is buzzy with a laid-back atmosphere that continues to the spacious rear pool terrace, which extends along a lengthy stretch of seafront and overlooks the sparkling blue waters of the Caribbean and the occasional enormous passing cruise ship.

Although this is an oceanfront property, the beach is man-made and small, which is a little bit of a let-down. It's nice enough, however, with white sand, straw umbrellas, and snorkeling just offshore -- but it lacks the sandy, zero-entry shores of the beaches in eastern Cozumel. While the Palace is family-friendly resort, clientele is mostly made up of couples, who spend their days sipping all-inclusive-plan cocktails on loungers around the pool or slipping off to spend their resort credits on island excursions or scuba diving trips.

Its best features are:

* Oceanfront resort with direct access to Caribbean Sea

* Within walking distance of San Miguel ferry port and nightlife

* Spacious rooms with large spa tubs, balconies, and sea views

* Two main pools with swim-up bar and very attentive poolside service

* Good selection of dining and round-the-clock room service

* Marble bathrooms have walk-in showers, quality toiletries, and bathrobes

* Concierge-level rooms include top-shelf liquor and luxury extras

Finally we decided to pack up our one lonely suitcase and get a taxi over to the Cozumel Palace. (We were a bit anxious to get home!) We were greeted with glasses of Champaign as we were registering at the desk. We were informed that our room was not yet ready but we were welcome to partake of any of the services offered. (bar, food, etc.)

As we were waiting to go to our room, we were offered whatever beverage we wished and asked to sit in the lobby to meet with a representative of the hotel. The Palace is a time share resort so we knew what to expect. The representative came over and presented his offer. Kathy asked if he was selling time shares and he said, "No, we don't call them time shares." We believe if it looks like a duck, quacks like a duck, it's likely a duck, and this was a duck! We politely decline; he approached us briefly one other time to which we gave him a stern no thank you and he never offered again throughout near our month long stay.

As we were relaxing in the lobby, another person approached us and inquired if we had any questions or concerns about anything to do with the hotel. I asked him about their gluten free food policy to which the gentleman replied, "I will get Head Waiter Luis for you. Luis approached us and assured me that they have many gluten free items on their menus and they often can adapt other menu items. During our stay, Luis went over the top to ensure I was eating safely; even to the point of going into the kitchen and bringing out gluten free desert items and other morsels of food for me.

A Promise Fulfilled

While in Cozumel we went on several adventures. On an early venture, we went to Diamonds International. Here Kathy met the "Pirate of her dreams!"

This store offered many styles of jewelry, including a pair of diamond rings that were the perfect pairing for Kathy's wedding ring. They embedded perfectly with her wedding ring and I allowed myself to be coerced by the sales staff while Kathy plied her bartering skills.

A Sinking Feeling!

Another adventure was quite exciting and educational. We went on the Atlantis Submarine and submerged one hundred plus feet in the Caribbean Sea to the second largest barrier reef system in the world, the Meso-American reef system, which spans almost 175 miles (280 km) of ocean between the Gulf of Mexico and Honduras. Cozumel's spectacular reef formations, effortless drift diving and exceptionally clear waters make this island one of the world's most popular diving destinations.

We were quite proud to learn the Atlantis is a Canadian owned company and the submarines are built in Canada.

Atlantis Submarines is a passenger submarine company. The company currently has 12 submarines and operates undersea tours in Grand Cayman, Barbados, Aruba, Guam, St. Thomas, Cozumel and in Hawaii at Kona, Maui and Oahu.

In order for passengers to reach the submarine they board a shuttle ferry, then they enter the submarine via steep stairs. When the submarine goes down they see corals, sunken ships, treasures, and fish through large viewports. When the submarine ride is finished the passengers are returned by the ferry to shore where they are given dive certificates. Some 12 million passengers have taken the Atlantis submarine tour to date.

The Atlantis XIV, which sails from Waikiki Beach, Hawaii, accommodates 64 passengers and is the world's largest passenger submarine.

Atlantis VII

Atlantis was founded by current president and CEO Dennis Hurd, a former designer of submersibles for North Sea oil rigs, with USD $3 million borrowed from friends and relatives. The company launched the world's first commercial passenger submarine tours in Grand Cayman in 1986.   Wikipedia

Scuttlebutt on the Jean Laffite

We were intrigued by the appearance of the pirate ship right from the get-go. We first saw it as we were landing; then again from our room at the Hotel Plaza. It was also a guide for us in the lost taxi!

We purchased tickets for the evening cruise which promised a fun evening including a dinner of steak or chicken with lobster tail. As we boarded the Jean Laffite they checked out our booty and had our photo taken with the crew.

We sat down on the wooden benches along the sides of the ship and were thoroughly entertained by the pirates. The grog kept coming continuously and we had to say no before becoming three sheets to the wind! Some people had done "terrible" things so they had to be punished doing games etc. You have to be a great sport, because you were centered out making people laugh etc.

After this was done, the pirates would make friends with you, hinting for some jewels etc.

We sailed for a short time then came out dinner, which the pirates prepared for us. The evening continued with music and dance. It was a great Pirate's of the Caribbean experience!

Bienvenido A Pepe's

Pepe's is a restaurant on the waterfront in downtown San Miguel two blocks from the main pier.

The menu offers cuisines of the world such as Asian, Italian and Mexican, without forgetting Angus Beef steaks and the seafood.

Kathy's long-time friend Joyce, who has a time share at the Cozumel Palace, was our guest for the evening. We enjoyed each other's company while relishing a delicious dinner of Angus steak and Caribbean lobster tail.

After dinner, we walked down Avenida Rafael E. Melgar to the area where we gathered to board the Jean Laffite. Because the area was under construction, Joyce was somewhat disappointed as she wanted to show us the church where every Sunday evening a crowd of locals would gather to sing gospel. We returned back to the hotel to retire for the evening.

All too soon it was time to go home and face the surgeon yet again. We arrived home on the 29th of February. We had two tasks in mind; empty the suitcases (which did show up three days after we arrived in Cozumel, apparently they went on their own vacation to Cancun!)

It was easier to read the mail than empty the suitcases so we did that first. Among the mound of mail was a letter from the surgeon stating that my February 4th appointment was rescheduled to February 11th. On February 11th, Kathy and I attended the surgeon's office and booked for surgery for March 5th. Already we're thinking, "We could have stayed in Cozumel for another month!"

Before March 5th arrived, we got as phone call from the surgeon's office to inform me that my surgery is being rescheduled for March 12th. On March 12th Kathy and I bravely made our way to the Health Sciences Center where I was registered and prepped for 10:00 o'clock surgery. By 11:30, I was still in the prep area with now word about when my surgery will be. Kathy inquired at the nurse's desk and was told it was delayed but could offer no details. Kathy decided to return home and I remained waiting. About 4:00 O'clock a nurse came in and told me my surgery had been cancelled and I would be rebooked.

The next morning I received a phone call from the surgeon's office. The person on the other end stated that, "Dr. S offers his sincere apologies; the cancelation of my procedure was inevitable. We are re-booking your surgery for March 17th and you will be the first surgery of the day." I thanked her for the phone call and felt assured that my next trip to HSC will actually be for the surgery.

Surgery day came and once again we bravely made our way to the HSC. Upon arriving we went to Admitting. We stepped up to the desk and gave the lady my name. She flipped through her files and stated, "You're not scheduled for surgery today Mr. Webster." I replied, "Are you sure?" She repeated, "You are not scheduled for surgery today."

I stepped back in and took a deep breath in an effort to remain calm. I then said to the clerk, "Let me tell you about our experience with this surgery. First of all, we came back early from our vacation in Mexico only to find out that we could have stayed for the planned two months. The surgery was scheduled for March 5th, and then rescheduled to March 12th. On March 12th I came in, was admitted, prepped and sat all day without food or water until 4 o'clock in the afternoon only to be sent home again. Now you are telling me I am not scheduled for surgery! I have had nine previous surgeries over the past twenty -three years and have never experienced such a miss managed mess!"

The clerk said, "I am very sorry for this, obviously there is a miscommunication here. I will make a couple of phone calls." Upon hanging up the phone, the clerk returned and said, "The Doctor's office failed to send us your file; you are scheduled for 9:00 this morning. Please return to the Surgeon's office and they will take you up to get prepped for surgery."

So, off we went and we were quickly whisked up to the pre-prep. I was given a gown and house coat and asked to get changed. I was told to leave my belongings in a locker and retain the key. After getting gowned up and ready, I returned to the waiting room. As we sat there I told Kathy that I felt something wasn't right with my belongings. We decided to inquire about it and sure enough I was mistaken for a day surgery patient; so the attendant went to my locker, out my belongings in the suit case and brought them back to my bed area.

As I was wheeled into the O.R. prep area, there was a swarm of O.R. staff milling about and as soon I appeared some of them came over to ask questions, put marks on me, etc. while the prep nurse was putting an intervenes in my hand. I was then taken into another room where the anesthesiologist attached an epidural. Then we were off to the O.R. Within minutes I was fast asleep and I don't recall much of what happened for the rest of the day. I awoke about 7:00 o'clock the next morning with no pain. I had two tubes projecting from my side plus the usual intravenous drip. I recovered as expected and on the following Monday the tubes were removed from my side and I was offered to be discharged that afternoon or the following morning, dependent on how I felt. Having spent so much time in hospitals, of which I am not a big fan, I opted for discharge that afternoon. I phoned Kathy and told her the good news and she came to help me get back home.

CHAPTER FOURTEEN

Mexican Misfortune

After the last surgery, I recovered as expected and quickly resumed our normal life. Part of our normal life is planning get-a-ways to warmer climates, usually in January. One of our favorite destinations is Mexico. We thoroughly enjoyed Cozumel and were there for one month. We had been to the east coast of Mexico twice now and now want to try the West coast so we began planning a trip to Puerto Vallarta. We prefer smaller resorts and our internet search pointed us to Dreams Puerto Vallarta Villa Magna. After much fact finding we booked this resort for January 2016.

In June, after having a C.T. Scan, I had a follow-up appointment with my surgeon. Again I was informed the scan shows a "spot" in my lung and they would follow this with another scan or x-ray in three months. In the meantime, he referred me to Cancer Care (CC) as they could not determine if the last cancer was lung cancer or if it metastasized from my colon or elsewhere.

Upon returning home from this appointment, I told Kathy about the spot and I said, "If I need more surgery, it will like happen late in the year or early next year and mess up our plans to go to Puerto Vallarta. We quickly decided to change our vacation date to late August to early September.

Kathy and I visited an oncologist at CC who was very professional and forthcoming. He explained my situation very well and informed us he was going to meet later that week with other oncologists and surgeons to discuss my case and then he would advise me of their recommendations.

On our next visit to CC, we were informed that the advisory council could not determine the source of my last tumor. He also told us the panel was unanimous that no further treatment such as chemotherapy is advised because of the adverse reaction I had from one dose in 2007. He also advised that my family doctor refer me to Dr. DI again to possibly continue with colonoscopies. I had not had one for several years because it was extremely difficult to start an IV. After having done one or two colonoscopies without any sedative, Dr. DI never scheduled any further tests and I never requested them.

On August 25th, we took to the air; going first to Toronto, then to Puerto Vallarta. We arrived at the Puerto Vallarta Airport and were quickly processed through Immigration and Security, and then we boarded the shuttle to go to the resort.

When we approached the resort, we drove up a steep drive way and stopped right in the middle of the hotel lobby! We stepped out of the shuttle and were greeted with "Welcome Home" and a sparkling glass of Champaign. Unbeknown to us, our travel agent, Lisa, tossed in a "Preferred Club Concierge" package so we were immediately taken to our room on the seventh floor. We requested a room near the elevator, which we got. The lobby on the seventh floor contained a self-help snack bar including alcohol. We simply just had to step out of our room for a snack or to go down to the main floor. Luckily for me, most of the "goodies" contained gluten so I wasn't enticed to "step out" frequently!

We were treated royally and enjoyed every moment of it. In spite of this, I ended up in the hospital for the last 2 or 3 days of our trip. It seems that I inadvertently got into some potato chips that contained gluten. I became dehydrated followed by a domino effect of other conditions. After the third day, the hotel doctor suggested I go to the hospital. At Amerimed, the doctor was concerned that my kidney may shut down. I was sent to I.C.U to be monitored while they flushed my system. Later I was returned to a regular patient room and by the next day was declared fit to fly and was discharged.

We made it to the airport just in time for our flight to Calgary! We overnighted in Calgary and arrived back home just in time for lunch!

On the following Saturday, we were to meet with family and friends for breakfast. When I woke up I was not feeling well again. I assumed that my kidneys may still be a problem and decided to go to the St. Boniface hospital Emergency to have it checked out. I took all the documents provided by the Amerimed Hospital.

After a short wait, I was taken into an E.R. Examination room. A nurse came in, checked my vitals and started an IV. After a while, a doctor came in and commented on the information provided from Amerimed. She did some tests which proved that my kidney was functioning normally so she sent me for a C.T. Scan. Apparently I had a partial obstruction in my stoma. This was a bit of a relief; a blockage can be cleared relatively easy to deal with whereas a kidney problem may become serious. I was admitted for a few days during which time my blockage cleared. During this visit, I was told the C.T. Scan also showed an aortic aneurysm and I was referred to a vascular surgeon.

In September, after getting a C.T. Scan, I had an appointment with the vascular surgeon. I used a wheel chair at this time as I was still quite weak from the events in Mexico and St. Boniface Hospital. Dr. B's description of my condition was very thorough and including the various surgical means at her disposal to correct the problem. My aneurysm measures 6.2 cm where as it normally measures 2.0 cm in the abdominal area. Surgery is recommended at 5.5cc. Obviously I am well into the recommended surgery zone but, because of so much scar tissue from previous surgeries, Dr. B can do only one procedure but does not recommend it. She stated, " A healthy thirty year old would take six months to recover from this procedure; given your medical history, you may not survive the surgery and if you do, it would likely take you well over a year to recover." That's one surgery I won't be having!

Abdominal aortic aneurysm (AAA), also known as a triple-a, is a localized enlargement of the abdominal aorta such that the diameter is greater than 3 cm or more than 50% larger than normal. They usually cause no symptoms except when ruptured. Occasionally there may be abdominal, back or leg pain. Large aneurysms can sometimes be felt by pushing on the abdomen. Rupture may result in pain in the abdomen or back, low blood pressure or a brief loss of consciousness.

AAAs occur most commonly in those over 50 years old, in men, and among those with a family history. Additional risk factors include smoking, high blood pressure, and other heart or blood vessel diseases. Genetic conditions with an increased risk include Marfan syndrome and Ehlers-Danlos syndrome. AAAs is the most common form of aortic aneurysm. Approximately 85 percent occur below the kidneys with the rest either at the level of or above the kidneys. In the United States screening males with ultrasound who are between 65 and 75 years old and have a history of smoking is recommended. In the United Kingdom screening all men over 65 is recommended. Australia has no guideline on screening. Once an aneurysm is found, further ultrasounds are typically done on a regular basis.

Not smoking is the single best way to prevent the disease. Other methods of prevention include treating high blood pressure, treating high blood cholesterol and not being overweight. Surgery is usually recommended when an AAA's diameter grows to >5.5 cm in males and >5.0 cm in females. Other reasons for repair include the presence of symptoms and a rapid increase in size. Repair may be either by open surgery or endovascular aneurysm repair (EVAR). As compared to open surgery, EVAR has a lower risk of death in the short term and a shorter hospital stay but may not always be an option. There does not appear to be a difference in longer term outcomes between the two. With EVAR there is a higher need for repeat procedures.

From Wikipedia

In a follow-up to the thoracic surgeon in October, I informed the surgeon's assistant about the events in the Amerimed Hospital, St. Boniface Hospital and about the aortic aneurism. When the surgeon entered the room, he threw his hands up into the air and declared, "What are we going to do with you!" He informed us the previous spot has not changed but there is another lesion "behind my larynx". This lesion appeared more formidable so I was scheduled to have another PET scan.

On December 7th, we visited the Oncologist who wanted to "keep in touch" as he had become our main support in dealing with all these issues. He asked me what I wanted to do about the situation I am now facing. I replied that," I know my time is limited and I want to maintain a quality of life. I want to be at home with Kathy and my family; not in hospitals and on operating tables. My one concern is that I am finding it takes me longer and longer to recover from surgeries, and if I have more cancer, should I have surgery, and if not, what will my life be like?" I was encouraged to try to take one day at a time and continue follow-up with the thoracic surgeon at this point in time.

I had the PET scan on November 24th, exactly eleven months since the first one. In mid-December, we visited the thoracic surgeon to learn the results of the scan. I have been seeing Dr. S since 2011 and have gotten to know him quite well. He is always polite and greets patients with a hand shake and a smile. When he has bad news, he will fumble and fiddle with your file or look on the computer. On this day, when we were fully expecting an announcement of more cancer, Dr. S came in with his usual smile and handshake, as did his assistant; but this time the smile remained as he said, "There is no cancer, go home and have a nice Christmas, we'll see you in three months!" There were smiles all around that day!

CHAPTER FIFTEEN

Another Triple Tragedy

Twenty fifteen did not end on a happy note. Kathy's Uncle Pat, (Dr. F.P. Doyle) after a long and fruitful life, passed away at the age of 93 years on December 2, 2015.

Just over three weeks later, our brother-in-law Ken, who, six months earlier was diagnosed with multiple myeloma was placed in palliative care just two weeks before his passing on December 24th. Once again I ask myself, "Why am I being spared?"

In April we received word of my cousin, Lynda Wright's passing on April 4th, 2016. On this occasion I was not able to attend the memorial due to problems with my ileostomy. Rest in Peace Lynda.

A Long deserved reprieve

Christmas happened again this year as it always does, with a few exceptions. We were invited to our niece Michelle and Dickson's new home which they had just purchased a few months earlier. It was a quiet Christmas, a somber mood prevailed.

My next appointment with the thoracic surgeon was looming and my expectations were not great. Finally in March, Kathy and I trotted off the see Dr. S., first stopping for an x-ray, then to his clinic. We waited for a few minutes, and then were called into the examination room. In reality, it was just a few minutes that we waited, but it seemed like an hour. Finally Dr. S came into the room and greeted us with his usual happy smile and handshake; He then turned to his computer and "pulled up" the x-ray taken that morning. He announced, "everything looks good, come back to see me in six months." We were elated!

So now we have a whole summer free of those pesky doctors and nurses, at least that's the hope. We may have to put up with pesky mosquitoes but we can swat them, you can't swat doctors and nurses!

I have decided to stop writing at this point and publish this book. I believe I have provided enough information that any self-respecting person with celiac disease cannot ignore thus will refrain from consuming gluten, in any amount and for any reason.

Food is, although somewhat more expensive, quite plentiful and available to everyone throughout the country. Folks who live in rural areas even have full access to gluten free food. Most people have computers and internet access and there are numerous businesses online that offer gluten free food products which they will ship anywhere in Canada. So I say to all celiac s "Please don't compromise your heath by eating gluten. Teach your children not to "cheat" on their gluten free diets, and watch them closely, especially as they approach their adolescent years.

Only you can prevent a life of many calamities and live a life of many celebrations!